Clinical Veterinary
Echography

Clinical Veterinary Echography

Federica Rossi

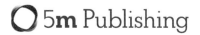 5m Publishing

First published 2013
This edition published by 5m Publishing 2017

Published by
5M Publishing Ltd,
Benchmark House,
8 Smithy Wood Drive,
Sheffield, S35 1QN, UK
Tel: +44 (0) 1234 81 81 80
www.5mpublishing.com

A Catalogue record for this book is available from the British Library

ISBN 978-1-910455-73-9

Book layout by Servis Filmsetting Ltd, Stockport, Cheshire
Printed by Replika Press Pvt Ltd, India
Photos and illustrations by Edizioni Veterinarie

Disclaimer:
To the extent permissible under applicable laws, no responsibility is taken by 5m
Publishing nor Edizioni Veterinarie for any injury and/or damage to persons or property
as a result of any actual or alleged libellous statements, infringements of intellectual
property, whether resulting from negligence or otherwise, or from any use or operation
of any ideas, instructions, procedures, products or methods contained in the material therein.

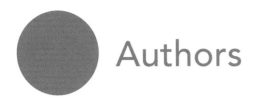

Authors

EDOARDO AURIEMMA

Edoardo graduated in Veterinary Medicine from the University of Parma in 2003. In 2003 he was 'laureato frequentatore' at the department of Clinical Medicine of the Faculty of Veterinary Medicine, Parma (Italy). He was visitor at the Diagnostic Imaging department, Faculty of Veterinary Medicine of Uppsala (Sweden) in 2004. From 2004 to 2008 he completed his Diagnostic Imaging residency at the Faculty of Veterinary Medicine of Utrecht (Netherlands), then in September 2008 he graduated from the European College of Veterinary Diagnostic Imaging (ECVDI). In 2005, Edoardo was visitor in the externship program of the Diagnostic Imaging department, Faculty of Veterinary Medicine, Knoxville (Tennessee). From September 2008 to November 2009 he was a contract employee at the Faculty of Veterinary Medicine of Utrecht. Currently he is a freelance radiologist at Istituto Veterinario di Novara and cooperates with several veterinary clinics as a diagnostic imaging adviser (teleradiology). He has authored and co-authored several publications on international journals. He is a speaker at a number of continuing education courses in diagnostic imaging for veterinary surgeons.

LUCA BENVENUTI

Luca graduated in Veterinary Medicine from the University of Pisa in 1998. Later, he ran continuing education workshops until 2000 with Dr. P. Barthez at the Ecole Vétérinaire of Lyon (France), Dr. G. Flaroutunian (freelance consultant in Veterinary Ultrasonography and Cardiology), and the 'Clinica Gran Sasso' with Dr. C. Bussadori (Dipl. ECVIM - Cardiology), mainly dealing with abdominal ultrasonography, and echocardiography. In 2000 he was awarded an eight-month fellowship in the Diagnostic Imaging department, Faculty of Veterinary Medicine, Liege (Belgium). From 2001 to 2005 he undertook part of the 'Training Programme' with an alternative schedule to obtain a diploma from European College of Veterinary Diagnostic Imaging (Prof. F. Snaps and Dr. V. Busoni, Dipl. ECVDI), also working as an intern at Paris and Lyon Ecole Vétérinaire. Since 2001 he has dealt with echocardiography and abdominal ultrasonography only, and carries out advisory services in Tuscany. He was a speaker at SVIDI (Società Veterinaria Italiana di Diagnostica per Immagini) Diagnostic Imaging Workshop, and taught courses on regional clinical ultrasonography (Sardinia and Apulia); since 2001 he has been a member of the European Association of Veterinary Diagnostic Imaging (EAVDI). He presented posters at EAVDI meetings in Murcia (Spain) in 2002 and Ghent (Belgium) in 2004. He co-authored the textbook *Medicina e chirurgia del coniglio da compagnia* published by Genoma (2012) on rabbit echocardiography. He is a speaker of the learning path in Diagnostic Imaging - Part II ('Ecografia base ed Ecografia Clinica') and a trainer at the SCIVAC course in advanced ultrasonography.

ELVANESSA CALERI

In 2005 Elvanessa graduated in Veterinary Medicine from the University of Pisa. In 2005–2006 she continuously attended the Clinica Valdinievole (PT). From 2006 to 2008, a grant let her carry out clinical and research work at the Diagnostic Imaging department of the University of Pisa. In December 2007, Elvanessa was a visitor at the Diagnostic Imaging department of the University of Zurich. In 2007 and 2008 she attended the Clinica dell'Orologio in Sasso Marconi (BO) and since 2009 she has collaborated with the same clinic, dealing with ultrasonography and radiology. Currently, she is a freelance vet professional in Tuscany and Emilia Romagna. She was a trainer in Diagnostic Imaging at the 2007 and 2008 Masters of Veterinary Oncology program at the University of Pisa. She is a speaker at the SCIVAC course in Clinical Ultrasonography.

GIAN MARCO GERBONI

Gian Marco graduated in Veterinary Medicine from the Faculty of Veterinary Medicine, University of Parma, in 1998. Since 1998 he had a one-year internship supervised by R.A. Santilli DVM Dipl. ECVIM-CA (Cardiology). Since 1999 he has worked at the Clinica Malpensa (VA) in charge of the Intensive Care Unit (ICU), dealing with internal medicine, first aid and abdominal ultrasonography. Also since 1999 he has dealt with scintigraphic studies and since 2006 with Interventional Radiology with an interest in the diagnosis and treatment of liver vascular abnormalities and ablative techniques of neoplastic injuries. He has been a trainer and a speaker at SCIVAC courses in Abdominal Ultrasonography, basic and advanced, since 2001. He was a speaker at the 2011 SCIVAC course in Advanced Emergency Medicine. He has authored papers in national and international veterinary journals. Since 2011 he has been SVIDI Vice President, and adviser of the Register of Veterinary Surgeons of Varese.

FEDERICA ROSSI

Federica graduated in November 1993 from the University of Bologna. Since 1993 she has specialized in Veterinary Radiology, and in 2003 she obtained a diploma from the European College of Diagnostic Imaging. She has authored more than 40 national and international scientific publications and revised Italian editions of some textbooks on Diagnostic Imaging; she also co-authored the *Radiologia del cane e del gatto (Poletto Editore)* textbook, the *BSAVA Manual of Canine and Feline Ultrasonography* (2011) and the *Veterinary Computed Tomography* textbook (ed. Wiley-Blackwell, 2011). From 2007 to 2009 she was President of the Società Veterinaria Italiana di Diagnostica per Immagini (SVIDI) and from 2006 to 2009 she was President of the European Association of Veterinary Diagnostic Imaging (EAVDI). Since 2010 she has President of SCIVAC. She has also been a freelance vet professional since 1993, carrying out advisory services in Diagnostic Imaging at Sasso Marconi (BO), where she deals in Radiology, Ultrasonography and Computed Tomography. She carries out research activities in the field of contrast enhanced ultrasonography.

She also works at the Centro Oncologico Veterinario (Sasso Marconi, BO), the first Italian Veterinary Radiotherapy centre, being one of the founding partners.

GILIOLA SPATTINI

In 1998 Giliola graduated in Veterinary Medicine with honours from the University of Parma.

In 1999 she won a post-graduate foreign grant and went to the Royal Veterinary College in London, where in 2000 she undertook a course at the European College of Diagnostic Imaging. She integrated her study plan with externships in the Universities of Utrecht, Uppsala, Tufts, Pennsylvania and Bern. In 2008 she obtained the European Diploma in Veterinary Diagnostic Imaging. In 2009 she completed her Ph.D. in the Diagnostic Imaging department at the University of Parma. She currently works at the Clinica Veterinaria Castellarano, in the Province of Reggio Emilia. She has authored national and international publications.

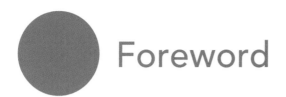

Foreword

This ultrasonography manual is designed as a useful tool for anyone willing to acquire the ultrasonographic methodology and/or to improve their level of acquisition and reading of ultrasonographic images.

This volume uses the experience of the SCIVAC Clinical Ultrasonography course; a ten-year tune-up took a group of speakers to grow together, optimizing their times, methods and teaching strategies so that they could transfer their theoretical/practical knowledge to participants.

The strong point of this manual is the practical, plain and schematic approach. The first few chapters summarize the accepted basis that followers of this methodology cannot ignore. Particular attention is given to ultrasound artefacts that even less experienced operators must recognize and understand. The fourth chapter is a key point of the manual, as it shows, through a number of pictures and diagrams, the basic steps to acquire a proper scanning technique and a systematic approach. Its special section includes a series of chapters dedicated to various abdominal and extra-abdominal organs. All chapters include a broad preamble with tables and diagrams that provide accurate guidelines to the identification of evaluated structures, and detailed information about normal ultrasonographic anatomy. The second part of each chapter in the special section is dedicated to ultrasonographic findings in any particular pathology; they are treated in a plain and schematic manner, with plenty of pictures.

We warmly thank all authors and friends, well beyond the conference rooms of Palazzo Trecchi, who made this manual a unique textbook. We hope it will be for many vets a valuable aid to be kept always close to their 'ultrasonographic device'.

Federica Rossi and Giliola Spattini
Sasso Marconi and Castellarano, March 2013

Acknowledgements

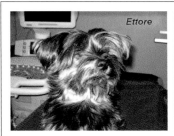

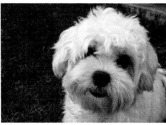

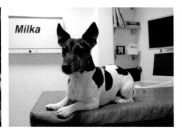

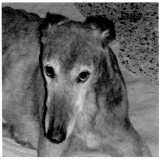

We would like to express a special thanks to people accredited for their input on this manual:

- Dott.ssa Elena Catania, Dott. Federico Gagliani, Dott. Carlo Anselmi
- Ettore, Mozzy, Playa, Milka and Jaga, for their great willingness during several ultrasonographic and photographic 'sessions'.
- Esaote group (Florence), for graphics cooperation.

I dedicate my work to 'Nonna Nina'.
Alzheimer's erased us from your memory, but never erased you from our hearts.

–Giliola Spattini

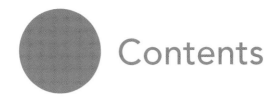

Contents

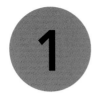

1 The physics behind ultrasounds

Giliola Spattini

FEATURES OF ULTRASOUNDS (Fig. 1.1)

Physical characteristics of ultrasounds	• Ultrasounds are mechanical oscillatory waves, so they require a propagation medium (Fig. 1.1a). • They do not propagate in a vacuum. • Propagation is via the compression and rarefaction of the material they contact with (Fig. 1.1b and 1.1c). • Oscillatory waves are characterized by frequency, wavelength and amplitude.
Frequency	• Frequency is the number of cycles within one second. • Hertz is the unit of frequency. A one kilohertz sound is equivalent to 1,000 cycles per second. • The human ear can perceive sounds up to 20,000 Hertz. • Ultrasonographic probes emit sounds with a frequency around 7,500,000 hertz, far above human hearing limits, hence the term 'ultrasounds'.
Wavelength	• Wavelength is the distance each cycle travels (λ) (Fig. 1.1a). • It is inversely proportional to the frequency. • The higher the frequency, the smaller the wavelength. • The smaller the wavelength, the higher the interactions with tissues passed through; hence the higher the frequency, the greater the resolution (Fig. 1.1d). • The more interactions occur, the more the ultrasound beam attenuates; hence the higher the frequency, the smaller the attainable scanning depth.
Amplitude (or intensity)	• Amplitude is the max variation in height of a periodic oscillation (A) (Fig. 1.1a). • It measures the level of compression and rarefaction applied to a tissue when an ultrasound crosses it. • To simplify matters, we can say it is the ultrasound energy, and only in this context we can identify it with the intensity. • The greater the amplitude, the higher the interactions with crossed tissues. • The amplitude of the ultrasound beam leaving the ultrasonographic probe is adjustable via the POWER button. • If the amplitude of the ultrasound beam is too high, the image will be saturated (too much echo, too low contrast, too white). • If the amplitude of the ultrasound beam is too low, the image spatial resolution and tissue penetration will be both very low.

ULTRASONOGRAPHIC PROBES (Fig. 1.2)

The ultrasonographic probe	• The ultrasonographic probe contains piezoelectric crystals that transform electric current into ultrasounds and vice versa. • It is the only part of the ultrasonographic device which comes into contact with the patient. • It emits ultrasounds for 1% of the time and receives them for 99% of the time. • It transforms ultrasounds reflected from tissues (which are called return echoes) into small electrical impulses that are analyzed by the computer unit. • Piezoelectric crystals are covered with a soft plastic that needs careful manipulation. • Never put the alcoholic solutions used to remove the skin lipid film in direct contact with the probe. • Once alcoholic detergents have evaporated from the patient's abdomen, the ultrasonographic gel can be applied and examination performed without risk to the probe.

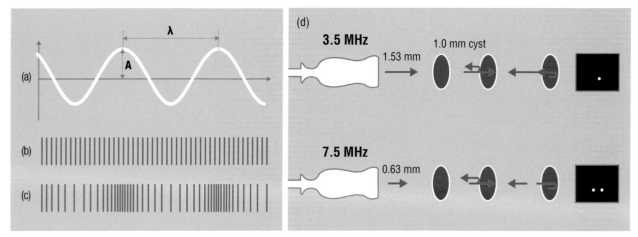

Figure1.1 a) Diagram of a mechanical wave. The distance a cycle travelled is the wavelength (λ). The maximum vertical variation is the amplitude (A). **b)** Schematic of an organic tissue before an ultrasound wave crossed it. **c)** An ultrasound is crossing an organic tissue: the tissue is compressed and rarefied by the energy of the propagating mechanical wave. **d)** An ultrasound beam typically includes three cycles. The cycle length is inversely proportional to the frequency: the higher the frequency, the shorter the ultrasound beam. For example, a 3.5 MHz frequency probe generates an ultrasound beam that is 1.53 mm in length. If the ultrasound beam runs into a cyst that is 1 millimetre in diameter, part of the beam is reflected at the first interface, while another part is reflected at the second interface. However, the cyst diameter is lower than the length of the ultrasound beam, so the two pulses merge and come back to the probe as a single echo. The monitor will show a point and the cyst will not be visible. A 7.5 MHz probe generates an ultrasound beam that is 0.63 mm in length. When this ultrasound beam runs into the same cyst, as previously seen, part of the beam is reflected at the first interface, while another part is reflected at the second interface. However, since the cyst diameter is greater than the echo length, the two ultrasounds will come back to the probe as two distinct points. Finally, the monitor shows the image of the cyst. These physical characteristics mean that the higher the ultrasound frequency, the greater the spatial resolution; nevertheless, due to smaller wavelength and major interactions with crossed tissues, the higher the frequency, the lower the penetration.

ULTRASONOGRAPHIC PROBES (Continued)

Linear probes	• Piezoelectric crystals are arranged in a linear pattern (Fig. 1.2a). • They generate a very limited near-field artefact (see Chapter 3, p. 17). • They generate images with the best axial and lateral resolution. • They require a large acoustic window. • Multifrequency probes are better suited to cover various patient sizes, preferably ranging between 7.5 and 13 MHz.
Microconvex probes	• Piezoelectric crystals are arranged in a semicircular pattern (Fig. 1.2b). • They require a small acoustic window. • They are the probes of choice for the cranial abdomen. • They are the most versatile probes for the abdomen of our patients, and give a good resolution/penetration trade-off. • Multifrequency probes ranging between 5 and 8 MHz are even better.
Sectoral or phased-array probes	• Piezoelectric crystals are arranged to make a square or rectangular surface (Fig. 1.2c). • They require a small acoustic window. • They feature an outstanding penetration and are the perfect probes for cardiology and thoracic ultrasonography. • They have poor lateral and axial resolution. • For cardiology of large breed dogs, best probes are in the 2.5–3.5 MHz range, while for cats and small breed dogs they are in the 5–7.5 MHz range.

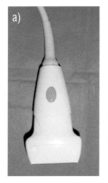
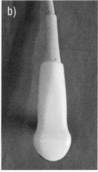
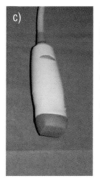

Figure 1.2 a) Linear probe: piezoelectric crystals are arranged in a linear pattern; this reduces the image deformation delivering the highest spatial resolution. **b)** Microconvex probe: crystals are arranged in a semicircle pattern so a small acoustic window is needed to obtain a wide line of vision. They have a limited spatial resolution compared to linear probes, but they are much more versatile. **c)** Sectoral probe: a small acoustic window is needed. Their ultrasonographic density is reduced compared to microconvex probes, but have better penetration and are excellent in evaluating moving organs. Not much useful for the abdomen, they are indispensable for cardiology.

ULTRASOUNDS PROPAGATION IN TISSUES (Fig. 1.3)

Acoustic impedance	• Acoustic impedance is the intrinsic resistance that a material offers to ultrasounds passage. • It affects their propagation speed in materials, and is directly proportional to the product of medium density and ultrasounds propagation speed in the medium itself. • $Z = v \times \rho$ • Z = acoustic impedance. • v = ultrasound speed in tissues. • ρ = density of crossed tissue. • Various biological tissues have slightly different impedances, and this is the principle of ultrasonography.

Acoustic impedance values in biological tissues	AIR	0.004	LIVER	1.65
	FAT	1.38	KIDNEY	1.62
	WATER	1.54	BLOOD	1.61
	BRAIN	1.58	BONE	7.80

Propagation speed values of ultrasounds in tissues	AIR	331 m/s	LIVER	1,549 m/s
	FAT	1,450 m/s	KIDNEY	1,561 m/s
	WATER	1,540 m/s	BLOOD	1,570 m/s
	BRAIN	1,541 m/s	BONE	4,080 m/s

Interface	• Pass-through points between tissues with different acoustic impedance are called interfaces. Whenever ultrasounds meet an interface, the beam is partially reflected (comes back) and partly propagated (absorbed from underlying tissues).
Propagation of ultrasounds in tissues with very similar acoustic impedance	• If an ultrasound crosses tissues with very similar acoustic impedances, it propagates in a linear mode and the image faithfully reproduces crossed anatomical structures (Fig. 1.3). • The ultrasound beam undergoes reflection (ultrasounds bounce back as echoes), propagation (it crosses the second tissue) and attenuation (being a mechanical wave, it dissipates energy as heat during its interactions with tissues).
Propagation of ultrasounds in tissues with very different acoustic impedance	• As they come at the interface of two materials with very different acoustic impedances, ultrasounds 'face a brick wall'. • A proportion of ultrasounds that is directly proportional to the difference in acoustic impedance of the second tissue is reflected back to the probe. • In interfaces where the second tissue has much lower acoustic impedance (e.g. colon wall and endoluminal gas content) (Fig. 1.3), the second tissue acts as very reflective material, causing the almost complete reflection of the ultrasound beam. • Only very few ultrasounds propagate in the tissue, and are then reflected back to the probe. • So, information is inadequate to obtain a diagnostic image of the second tissue. A dirty posterior acoustic shadow is created (see Chapter 3, p. 17). • In interfaces where the second tissue has a higher acoustic impedance (e.g. intestinal wall and endoluminal foreign body), the second tissue acts as highly absorbent tissue; so a small percentage of ultrasounds is reflected by the interface, but most of them are propagated (in concrete terms, they are absorbed by the tissue). • The difference in acoustic impedance prevents ultrasounds being reflected back to the probe. • The second tissue does not reflect echoes. • Again, a posterior acoustic shadow is created, but it is called 'clean' (see Chapter 3, p. 17).

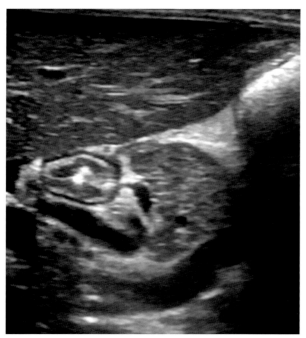

Figure 1.3   Propagation of ultrasounds through tissues with very similar acoustic impedance. In this feline patient, we can locate the liver, the duodenum, the right pancreatic lobe, the portal vein, the dilated common cystic duct, and the colon. Acoustic impedances are very similar, hence ultrasounds propagate in a linear manner. Distally to the colon instead, intraluminal gas has very different acoustic impedance, so a 'dirty posterior acoustic shadow' artefact is visible. Due to this artefact, a diagnostic image cannot be obtained from tissues distal to the colon.

PRODUCTION OF ULTRASONOGRAPHIC IMAGES (FIG. 1.4)

The computer	• The computer receives electrical impulses from return echoes processed by the probe. • It transforms small electrical impulses into images. • It uses postulates, i.e. rules considered always true.
Postulates	• The probe emits a single ultrasound beam. • Ultrasounds always travel in a straight line. • Return echoes (ultrasounds reflected from tissues) are raised from structures located on the longitudinal axis of ultrasound beam. • The ultrasound speed in tissues is constant, the ultrasounds received later by the transducer are those reflected from deeper structures. • The intensity of the return ultrasound is directly proportional to characteristics of the reflective tissue.
Spatial reconstruction of images	• The postulates 1, 2 and 3 define the position of echoes on the X axis (Fig. 1.4a). • The postulate 4 defines the position of echoes on the Y axis (Fig. 1.4b). • The postulate 5 defines the echogenicity of the reflected ultrasound (Fig. 1.4c).

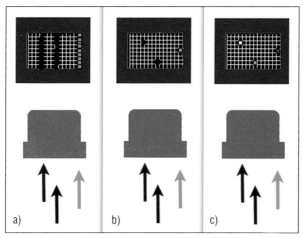

Figure 1.4   a) The computer is based on the postulate that ultrasounds always travel in a straight line. This way, simply analyzing the echo entry point, return echoes can be placed in the correct lateral position.

b) The computer is based on the postulate that ultrasounds travel at constant speed; so the echo can be placed on the Y plane, considering the time spent to come back to the probe: echoes that come back later are the deeper ones.

c) The computer is based on the postulate that intensity of reflected ultrasounds is only related to properties of tissues that reflected them: so their echogenicity is easy to define.

THE PHYSICS BEHIND THE DOPPLER EFFECT (FIG. 1.5–7)

Christian Johann Doppler (1803–1853)	• An Austrian mathematician and physicist, he was the first to mathematically describe the effect, hence the name. • Think of an ambulance siren sound: the sound seems to be higher in intensity when it is approaching. When the ambulance is receding the sound seems to get lower and lower. However, the ambulance siren sound is constant in intensity. • The different perception of sound if the source is approaching or receding is called Doppler effect.
The physics behind the Doppler effect	• If a receiver is going closer to a sound source, reflected echoes have higher acoustic frequency (Fig. 1.5a) • If a receiver is moving away from a sound source, reflected echoes have lower acoustic frequency (Fig. 1.5b).
Mathematical formula of the Doppler effect	$$f_d = \frac{V \times 2(f_0) \times \cos \alpha}{C}$$ • f_d = the Doppler shift or the frequency change due to the Doppler effect. • V = the speed of the receiver or the evaluated blood flow. • f_0 = the frequency of the incident sound or the ultrasound emitted from the ultrasonographic probe. • $\cos \alpha$ = the angle of incidence between ultrasound beam and receiver. • C = the sound speed in tissues.
$$V = \frac{f_d \times C}{2(f_0) \times \cos \alpha}$$	• The mathematical formula of the Doppler effect can be used to compute the speed of blood flow. • The formula shows that the determinant is the angle of incidence, as if the blood vessel is parallel to the ultrasound beam, the cosine of zero degrees is equal to 1, so we will have the maximum measurement of the blood flow; on the contrary, if the ultrasound beam is perpendicular to the vessel, we will have no detectable blood flow since the cosine of 90 degrees is equal to zero.
Visualization of the Doppler effect	• With the Doppler effect, the frequency of return echoes is compared with the frequency of the original sound. • This difference is called Doppler shift. • This difference is in the kilohertz range, so it's audible to the human ear and is transformed into sound. • You can view the Doppler effect in form of coloured pixels superimposed over the image: Colour Doppler and Power Doppler are displayed this way. • The information can be shown in a Cartesian system, with the time put on the horizontal axis and the Doppler shift on the vertical axis: Continuous Wave (CW) Doppler, and Pulsed Wave (PW) Doppler are displayed this way.
Colour Doppler	• This yields a colour map linked to the Doppler shift and superimposed on a two-dimensional image (Fig. 1.6). • It identifies the presence and direction of a blood flow within a selected area. • It provides general information about blood flow that is only subjectively evaluable, not numerically quantifiable. • By convention, echoes reflected from a blood flow and approaching the probe are represented with red pixels. • Echoes reflected from a blood flow and moving away from the probe are represented with blue pixels.
CW (Continuous Wave) Doppler	• This system emits and receives ultrasounds without interruption. • A crystal emits ultrasounds and a different crystal receives them. • It receives and encodes all blood flows in a selected scan plane, adding them together. • It shows the total speed and direction of flows added together. • It cannot identify the speed or the direction of a specific blood vessel within the scan plane. • It can measure high speeds and is the method of choice in cardiology (Fig. 1.7a).
PW (Power Wave) Doppler	• The same crystal sends impulses first, then receives them. • It provides information about speed and direction of a blood flow located at a preselected specific point. • The area you want to receive the signal from can be changed. • It can only measure low-capacity blood flows, generally below 2 m/s, so it is not suitable for cardiology (Fig. 1.7b).

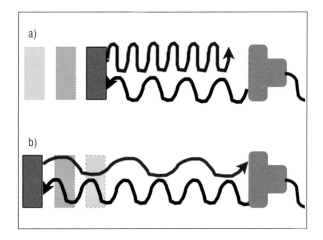

Figure 1.5 a) An ultrasound beam strikes an approaching object: the frequency of return echoes increases. **b)** An ultrasound beam strikes an object moving away: the frequency of return echoes decreases.

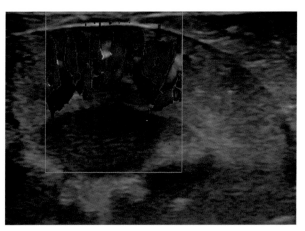

Figure 1.6 Imagine the Colour Doppler applied to a two-dimensional image of a feline kidney. The Colour Doppler identifies the blood flow within renal vessels, based on the Doppler shift. Red coloured vessels have a positive Doppler shift, so they generated return echoes with higher frequency compared to ultrasounds emitted by the probe: it means the vessel's blood flow is approaching the probe. Blue coloured vessels have a negative Doppler shift, so they generated return echoes with lower frequency compared to ultrasounds emitted by the probe: it means the vessel's blood flow is moving away from the probe.

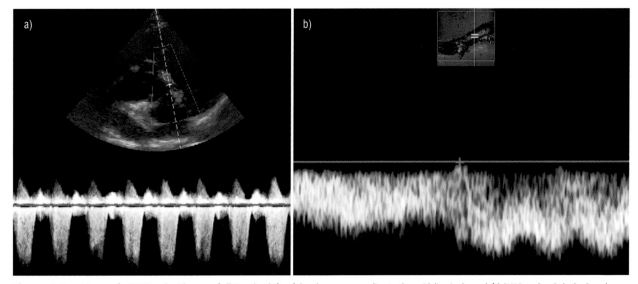

Figure 1.7 a) Image of a CW Doppler. The sum of all Doppler shifts of the plane corresponding to the guideline is showed. **b)** PW Doppler. Only the Doppler shift of the area within a sampling volume is showed. In this case, it is the core of the evaluated vessel.

RECOMMENDED READING

Wells PN, Liang HD, Young TP: Ultrasonic imaging technologies in perspective. J Med Eng Technol. 2011, Aug-Oct; 35(6–7): 289–299.

Coltrera MD: Ultrasound physics in a nutshell. Otolaryngol Clinic North Am. 2010, 43(6): 1149–1159.

Wood MM, Romine LE, Lee YK, Richman KM, O'Boyle MK, Paz DA, Chu PK, Pretorius DH: Spectral doppler signature waveforms in ultrasonography: a review of normal and abnormal waveforms. Ultrasound Q. 2010, Jun; 26(2): 83–89.

Bushberg JT, Seibert JA, Leidholdt EM, Boone JM: Ultrasound. In: Bushberg JT, Seibert JA, Leidholdt EM, Boone JM: The Essential Physics of Medical Imaging. Williams & Wilkins, second edition, 2002, 469–555.

Kremkau FW: Physics of Ultrasound. In Kremkau FW: Diagnostic ultrasound: principles and instruments. WB Saunders Co, sixth edition, 2002, 273–311.

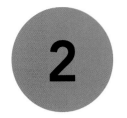

2 Fundamentals of ultrasonographic images interpretation

Giliola Spattini

FUNDAMENTALS OF ULTRASONOGRAPHIC IMAGES INTERPRETATION (Fig. 2.1–5)

Criteria to assess in each ultrasonographic image	• As with any diagnostic imaging method, ultrasonography also is based on well-defined criteria and specific terminology. Each ultrasonographic image must be evaluated for:

LOCATION	EDGES
MORPHOLOGY	ECHOSTRUCTURE
RELATIONS WITH OTHER ORGANS	ECHOGENICITY
SIZE	NUMBER
SHAPE	

Location	• The position occupied by evaluated structure. The most commonly used terminology is:
	  – Within normal limits: this terminology is preferred to 'normal' since determining whether an organ is really normal is difficult and very subjective.
	  Consider the renal corticomedullary differentiation in a 13-year-old patient: it is very commonly reduced. This ultrasonographic sign will not receive much clinical weight; however, it is not 'normal' but within normal limits for a 13-year-old patient.
	  – Dislocated: an organ that moved from its original site. Often, spleen and kidneys are dislocated dorsally by large masses originating from the ventral abdomen.
	  – Rotated: a structure that is turning around its own axis or around another body ends up going upside down. Sometimes, the splenic hilum is placed dorsally compared to parenchyma. The spleen is a relatively movable organ, so it can rotate in the abdomen, especially at the spleen tail.
	  – Torsion: an organ wraps around itself, leading to the narrowing of areas on the tributary vascular system with serious clinical consequences. Most common abdominal torsions are the gastric torsion (not usually an ultrasonographic diagnosis, but clinical and radiographical), the splenic torsion and the testicular torsion (more common in cryptorchids).
	• Another parameter is the distribution of a pathological process that can be:
	  – Localized: delimited in space, e.g. a pathological process in a single liver lobe.
	  – Focal: one and only localized injury.
	  – Multifocal: several well-defined injuries.
	  – Diffuse: the whole organ is affected by the pathological process.

Morphology	• The physical appearance of a structure, i.e. elements that make it recognizable as an organ
	  – Within normal limits.
	  – Preserved: maintained; despite changes in echostructure and echogenicity, the evaluated organ is still identifiable.
	  – Altered: changed; the original organ is still identifiable, but different from the norm; e.g. because some nodules alter its edges, or because components that make up the organ changed.
	  – Destroyed: totally altered, so the appearance of the original organ is lost. Usually, relationships with surrounding organs are changed as well.
	  – Unrecognized: some organs are not identifiable, due to their physical (size) or ultrasonographic (isoechoic compared to surrounding tissues) characteristics. Pathological processes can change an organ morphology making it unrecognizable. This often occurs with large abdominal masses, where the original organ of a mass can be very difficult or impossible to identify by ultrasonography only.

FUNDAMENTALS OF ULTRASONOGRAPHIC IMAGES INTERPRETATION (Continued)

Relation with other organs	• How different structures interface with each other: – Adjacent: two organs that are very close and in contact but seem to be disconnected; e.g. because they do not move in sync during breaths. – Tight: two very close organs that move in sync: they can be hard to evaluate, especially with abdominal masses. – Infiltrated and/or impinged: a pathological process that extends to another organ. Example: an adrenal carcinoma that partially occludes the caudal vena cava through the phrenicoabdominal vein.
Size	• The volume of the evaluated organ: – Within normal limits. – Increased: there are no reference measurements for all abdominal organs; sometimes, as with the liver size, the evaluation is subjective. – Decreased: there are no reference measurements for all abdominal organs; sometimes, as with the liver volume, the evaluation is subjective.
Shape	• The outer profile of an organ, i.e. its conformation: – Preserved: maintained; a lymph node can be very enlarged while keeping its oval shape. – Altered: a nodule that deforms the pole cranial edge of an adrenal gland alters the gland shape. – Rounded: an organ may be more rounded than expected. – Oval: in some organs, a change in shape is one of the most significant features of active disease. Example: an oval lymph node that gets rounded, notably in combination with increased size, can be easily indicative of neoplastic infiltration.
Edges	• The organ limits, its ends (Fig. 2.1): – Within normal limits. – Within normal limits. – Regular: if they are linear, without concavities or convexities. – Irregular: if they have concavities and convexities. – Rounded: e.g. in a liver with hepatomegaly. – Sharp: e.g. a reduced liver with the parenchyma within normal limits. – Well-defined: if easily followed and differentiated from surrounding tissues. – Ill-defined: for example, an end-stage kidney that is poorly defined compared to surrounding tissues. – Unidentifiable: for example, if the organ seems to continue without interruption into a pathological process; two very close structures could not generate identifiable edges.
Echogenicity	• The properties of a tissue to generate echoes. • Relative echogenicity: the echogenicity of the evaluated organ compared to the echogenicity of adjacent organs. • Common terminology (Fig. 2.2): – Anechoic with posterior-wall enhancement: a structure that does not generate reflected echoes and attenuates the ultrasound beam to a lesser extent compared to soft tissues, due to its lower density. So, distally to the anechoic tissue, the other tissues will be most echoic compared to adjacent ones (see Chapter 3, p. 17). This is almost always associated with fluid collections. – Anechoic: a tissue that does not generate reflected echoes and appears completely black, typical of necrotic tissues. – Hypoechoic: a tissue that generates less return echoes compared to reference tissues, and that typically appears dark grey in the final image. – Isoechoic: a tissue that generates the same return echoes compared to reference tissues. – Echoic: a tissue that generates a good number of return echoes and appears light grey in the final image. – Hyperechoic: a tissue that generates many return echoes compared to reference tissues and is usually very light grey or white in the final image. – Hyperechoic with a posterior acoustic shadow: a tissue with almost-white interface, greater density compared to soft tissues, and that absorbs ultrasounds thus creating a completely black acoustic shadow below the interface. This is typical of foreign bodies and bone tissue. • Factors affecting the echogenicity: – Content of water: the more the water, the less echoic the tissue. – Content of connective tissue: the more the connective content, the more echoic the tissue.

FUNDAMENTALS OF ULTRASONOGRAPHIC IMAGES INTERPRETATION (Continued)

Echogenicity	• In order from the more anechoic to the more hyperechoic we see:

1) BILE, URINE	5) LIVER
2) RENAL MEDULLARY	6) DEPOT FAT
3) MUSCLE	7) SPLEEN
4) RENAL CORTEX	8) PROSTATE

	• The tissues' echogenicity changes depending on the probe frequency, so two tissues must be compared using the same probe at the same frequency.

Echostructure
Figs. 2.3, 2.4, 2.5
	• Features of single echoes that, overall, make up the texture of the evaluated structure.
	• Size of dots that make up the texture:
	  – Fine (small pixels) (Fig. 2.3).
	  – Intermediate (mean pixels) (Fig. 2.4).
	  – Coarse (large pixels) (Fig. 2.5).
	• Another echostructure key element is the homogeneity:
	  – Homogeneous: the whole organ has the same echostructure.
	  – Not homogeneous: the same organ has different echostructures.

Number	• Counting injuries and organs is recommended, when possible. The common terminology is:
	  – Within normal limits.
	  – Increased: for example, if an accessory spleen is seen.
	  – Decreased: for example, renal agenesis and only one kidney visible on ultrasonography.

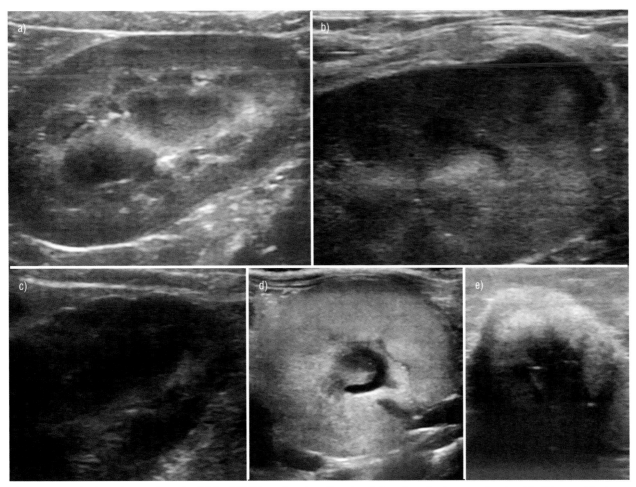

Figure 2.1   **a)** Kidney edges, regular and well-defined. **b)** Kidney edges altered by an isoechoic neoformation that warps the edge of the kidney caudal pole. Edges are well-defined. **c)** Kidney edges are irregular and tend to be wavy, instead of smooth and regular. They are also less defined compared to the norm. **d)** Edges are regular but less defined compared to the norm. **e)** Edges are irregular and ill-defined

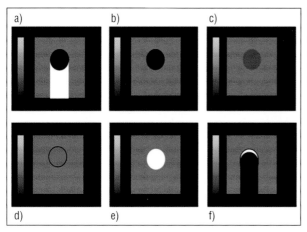

Figure 2.2 **a)** Anechoic structure with posterior-wall enhancement, typical of fluid collections. **b)** Anechoic structure without posterior-wall enhancement, typical of necrotic structures. **c)** Hypoechoic structure compared to surrounding tissues. **d)** Isoechoic structure compared to surrounding tissues. **e)** Hyperechoic structure compared to surrounding tissues. **f)** Hyperechoic interface structure with clean posterior shadowing.

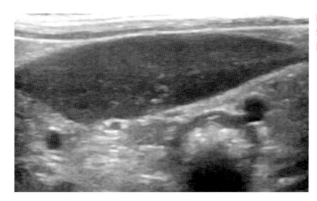

Figure 2.3 Spleen, an organ with fine echostructure. The splenic texture seems to be made by very fine uniform pixels, hence the regular and homogeneous parenchyma appearance.

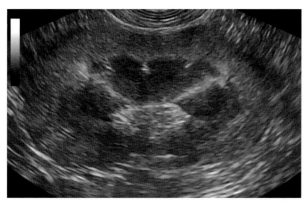

Figure 2.4 The renal cortex has an intermediate echostructure. Pixels are larger and less uniform compared to those of the spleen. However, the final appearance of the renal cortex remains homogeneous.

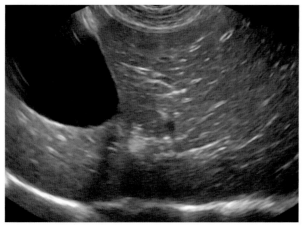

Figure 2.5 Liver, a typical organ with coarse echostructure. Pixels are large and different from each other, generating a non-uniform texture. This echostructure is typical of the liver.

THE ULTRASONOGRAPHIC REPORT (Fig. 2.6)

The ultrasonographic report	• The report must include the identification of facility/veterinary surgeon, patient's owner and patient, the signalment and the history. • It must include a descriptive part to detail evaluated organs, using the ultrasonography jargon. • It must show which organs have been assessed and which were not. • The description must allow a colleague to draw assessed organs, even without images available. • It must include a section for the ultrasonographic diagnosis, where injuries considered significant are indicated. • It must have a list of differential diagnoses, from the most likely to the least likely, with the features that led to order them in such a way. • It must have the conclusions, i.e. what the ultrasonographer read in images based on signalment, history and lab tests. • It can include advice on possible second steps (biopsies, second level of diagnostic imaging [CT, MRI], surgery).
Example: Identification	• IDENTIFICATION, SIGNALMENT, HISTORY **SURGERY/CLINIC/VETERINARY HOSPITAL XXX** Health Manager: xxxxx xxxxxx Address xxxx Owner: _____ Date: _____ / _____ **ABDOMINAL ULTRASOUND REPORT** Species: DOG/CAT Breed: Sex: M MC FS F Name: Age: Referent Dr: Anamnesis: • Example: Lillo, 8-year-old Persian cat, presented with polyuria and polydipsia. Slight rise in kidney parameters; abnormalities found on kidneys; palpation required a urinary-tract ultrasonographic examination (Fig. 2.6)
Descriptive part	• KIDNEY: Bilaterally, there are some oval or rounded structures in the cortex and medullary (Fig. 2.6) These injuries warp echostructure and renal morphology, distorting edges. Structures have anechoic content and show posterior-wall enhancement. The content remains anechoic, even using higher values for power and gain. These structures are bounded by a thin, regular and uniform echoic wall. There is not much undamaged renal parenchyma. The vascularization is very limited in anechoic structures, and reduced in the kidney hilum area. There is a slight dilation of the left renal pelvis that does not exceed 2.1 mm. There is no associated hyperechogenicity of peripelvic tissues.
Ultrasonographic diagnosis	• Severe impairment of renal morphology due to multiple uncomplicated renal cysts.
Differential diagnoses	• PKD. • Very unlikely, multiple renal cysts non-genetic but degenerative in nature. • An infiltrative pathology is very unlikely due to poor vascularization of injuries and posterior-wall enhancement.
Comments	• Given signalment, clinical picture, lab tests and ultrasonographic images, the active pathology is compatible with a polycystic kidney disease, probably genetic in nature. • Kidney images may raise a suspicion of chronic renal failure to be confirmed by lab tests.
Further diagnostic evaluations suggested	• Blood tests, biochemical panel and urinalysis to specify if the patient is in renal failure, failure degree included. • Genetic evaluation of the subject for PKD, notably if a predisposed breed, and if the subject is genetically related to a set of ancestors used for breeding.
Signature of veterinary sonographer	• IDENTIFICATION: – The name of veterinary sonographer must be readable and identifiable. – It is fine to add a phone number in case a colleague needs further clarification.

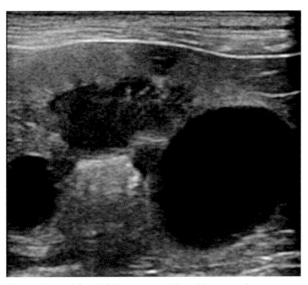

Figure 2.6 Polycystic kidney in a cat; PKD-positive at genetic tests.

RECOMMENDED READING

Duszak R, Nossal M, Schofield L, Picus D: Physician documentation deficiencies in abdominal ultrasound reports: frequency, characteristics, and financial impact. J Am Coll Radiol. 2012, Jun; 9(6): 403–408.

Ihnatsenka B, Boezaart AP: Ultrasound: Basic understanding and learning the language. Int J Shoulder Surg. 2010, Jul; 4(3): 55–62.

Eze KC, Marchie TT, Eze CU: An audit of ultrasonography performed and reported by trainee radiologists. West Afr J Med. 2009, Jul-Aug; 28(4):257–261.

Sutherland T: Demystifying abdominal ultrasound. Aust Fam Physician. 2009, Oct; 38(10): 797–800.

Le T, Fayadh RA, Menard C, Hicks-Boucher W, Faught W, Hopkins L, Fung-Kee-Fung M: Variation in ultrasound reporting on patients referred for investigation of ovarian masses. J Obstet Gynaecol Can. 2008, Oct; 30(10): 902–906.

3 Artefacts in ultrasonography

Giliola Spattini

In ultrasonography, an artefact is 'everything that is not representative of the evaluated structure, but is temporary'.
Artefacts may:

- Give a real appearance to nonexistent structures
- Do not allow the visualization of some structures
- Increase or decrease the echogenicity of the region of interest
- Alter shape and size of a structure in the final ultrasonographic image.

Origin of the most commonly observed artefacts			
Environmental	**Operator-dependent**	**Ultrasounds–patient interaction**	**Artefacts generated by the ultrasonographic device**
Electromagnetic artefacts	Poor patient's preparation	Repetition	Near-field artefact
	Excessive probe tilt compared to the tissue	Reverberation and comet tail	Artefact from wrong evaluation of propagation speed
	Wrong settings on the ultrasonographic device	Ring-down	Posterior-wall enhancement
		Posterior acoustic shadow	Partial-volume artefact
		Mirror effect	Side-lobe artefacts
		Refraction	

OBSERVED ARTEFACTS

Environmental artefacts:	**CAUSE:** • An electromagnetic interference that produces luminous bands or glares, pulsed or uninterrupted.
Electromagnetic artefacts (Fig. 3.1)	**PRESENTATION:** • A series of luminous points flow in an orderly way over the image, forming rain, network or wave effects (Fig. 3.1) • They appear independently from the contact between probe and patient. **HOW TO REDUCE/PREVENT THEM:** When possible, identify the interfering equipment (medical electrical equipment, air-conditioners, hair-clippers) and switch it off during the ultrasonographic examination.
Operator-dependent artefacts	**CAUSE:** • The air in contact with the probe surface prevents the ultrasounds propagation and acquisition of proper images from the patient.
Poor preparation of the acoustic window	• Plenty of air trapped between hair locks. Remove it consistently. • It is recommended to degrease the skin surface with alcohol to remove dirt and impurities that can hamper the ultrasounds transmission. • Even crusts or mud encrustations hinder the correct passage of ultrasounds and strongly degrade the image. **PRESENTATION:** • Images are too dark and poor of reflected echoes; echostructures are coarse, edges are undefined.

OBSERVED ARTEFACTS (Continued)

Poor preparation of the acoustic window	**HOW TO REDUCE/PREVENT THEM:** • Plenty of gel is applied to the shaved and cleaned patient's skin; this removes the air and moisturises the skin, allowing for a better transmission of the ultrasound beam. • In very dehydrated patients and some Nordic breeds the skin is less suited to ultrasounds passage, so it is necessary to thoroughly degrease it and apply some gel 15 minutes before the exam.
Excessive probe tilt compared to evaluated structure	**CAUSE:** • Excessive tilt of the ultrasonographic probe compared to the evaluated structure prevents return echoes to reach piezoelectric crystals, thus creating a poorly detailed image. **PRESENTATION:** • Structures with different homogeneity show focal hypoechoic areas with coarse echostructure. • This artefact is notably visible with linear probes. **HOW TO REDUCE/PREVENT THEM:** • If the hypoechoic area is really an injury, it must appear in two orthogonal scan planes at least, persisting even after moderate probe tilts. • The probe must be placed as perpendicular as possible to the evaluated structure.
Wrong settings made by the operator on the ultrasonographic device	**CAUSE:** • Power and gain settings too high or too low. • Power: the amplification of outgoing ultrasound beam. • Gain: the amplification of ultrasound echoes coming back from tissues. **PRESENTATION:** • Too high power and gain settings saturate the image: all tissues are hyperechoic and not contrasted enough (Fig. 3.2) • Too low power and gain settings generate an image where all tissues are hypoechoic, with coarse texture. **HOW TO REDUCE/PREVENT THEM:** • There is a tendency to increase power a lot when the ultrasonography environment is too well lit or the patient skin not properly prepared. • A good trade-off is setting power to 75% and gain to 50%. • These parameters may vary from one ultrasonographic device to another.

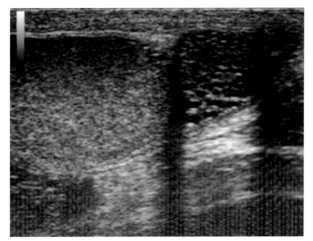

Figure 3.1 Electromagnetic artefact with rain effect. The image shows a testicle and its epididymis. Adapted from: Spattini G: Gli artefatti in ecografia veterinaria: come riconoscerli e correggerli. Veterinaria, 22(1): 9–20, 2008.

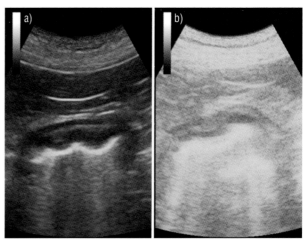

Figure 3.2 **a)** Image with correct power and gain settings (stomach). **b)** Image with wrong power and gain settings. Both are too high and the image is saturated, losing contrast and grayscale.

OBSERVED ARTEFACTS

Artefacts due to ultrasounds–patient interaction **Repetition (Fig. 3.3a)**	**CAUSE:** • The gas has very low acoustic impedance. • This is why at the soft tissues–gas interface almost all ultrasounds of the main beam are reflected back toward the probe, and only a few are able to propagate in tissues. • So, the primary beam comes back to the probe at the same time. • The probe cannot absorb the primary beam that comes back from tissues, hence acting as highly reflective tissue and throwing back all the primary beam to the soft tissues–gas interface. The cycle repeats until the primary beam is entirely depleted, due to the energy dispersion required by propagation between the highly reflective interface and the probe. **PRESENTATION:** • A series of parallel hyperechoic lines is generated; they recur at intervals that are a multiple of the distance between the probe and the highly reflective interface (Fig. 3.3a). • The interval between a hyperechoic line and the next one is the time the ultrasound beam takes to reach the reflective interface and come back to the probe. **HOW TO REDUCE/PREVENT THEM:** • Whenever there is a united front of gas, such as in the pulmonary interface, this artefact can not be avoided.
Reverberation (Fig. 3.3b) and comet tail (Fig. 3.3c)	**CAUSE: REVERBERATION** • With a repetition artefact, if the highly reflective acoustic surface is irregular and surrounded by tissues with different acoustic impedance, multiple reflections are created within the highly reflective interface and extra-echoes are produced; their distance is not a multiple of the distance between the probe and the interface and this is called reverberation. **CAUSE: COMET TAIL** • With a reverberation artefact, if the highly reflective acoustic surface is very small (gas bubbles) and included in tissues with very different acoustic impedance, multiple reflections are created within the highly reflective interface, producing extra-echoes so close that they merge together. **PRESENTATION:** • The REVERBERATION shows a series of moderately sized hyperechoic parallel lines, interspersed with uneven hyperechoic echoes (Fig. 3.3b). The distance between these lines is not a multiple of the distance between the reflecting surface and the probe. • The COMET TAIL appears as a series of very thin hyperechoic lines, very close together, almost merged, that fade away with increasing depth (Fig. 3.3c). It is uneven and very mobile, and follows the movement of the small air bubble that generates it. **HOW TO REDUCE/PREVENT THEM:** • They are impossible to reduce or prevent, but are useful to detect free air; they can show abdominal free air, an abscess or a mass (if the mass is abdominal and contains air, its intestinal origin is very likely). • The 'comet tail' artefact must be differentiated from another called ring-down, and from artefacts created by small metallic foreign bodies. **CAUSE: ARTEFACTS FROM SMALL METALLIC FOREIGN BODIES** • They have a high acoustic impedance compared to surrounding soft tissues, so they usually create a highly reflective interface and clean posterior acoustic shadow. • When they are very small and unable to absorb all ultrasounds, they behave as highly reflective tissues and throw back the entire ultrasound beam to the probe. **PRESENTATION:** • If they are very small, they create a reverberation or a comet tail. • They differ from a gas-generated comet tail because while the former is uneven and movable, the artefact caused by a small metallic foreign body is even and constantly static (Fig. 3.4). • If doubts persist, make an X-ray. **HOW TO REDUCE/PREVENT THEM:** • This artefact cannot be avoided, but must be used to identify a small metallic foreign body.

OBSERVED ARTEFACTS (Continued)

Ring-down (Fig. 3.5)	**CAUSE:** • It appears when very small gas bubbles in polyhedral formation enclose a small fluid collection. • The centre acts as a resonance box and generates ultrasounds as if it was a piezoelectric crystal. **PRESENTATION:** • Echoes are vertical and not horizontal as in the comet tail. • It is more intense and expands more in the deep than on the surface; it fans out (Fig. 3.5). **HOW TO REDUCE/PREVENT THEM:** • The ring-down cannot be avoided, but many ring-down artefacts on a diaphragmatic interface must raise a suspicion of excessively high content of alveolar fluid, i.e. a pulmonary oedema.
Posterior acoustic shadow (Fig. 3.6–7)	**CAUSE:** • Highly reflective (gas, air) or highly attenuating materials (bones, foreign bodies) cause a lack of echoes reflected from underlying tissues, hence creating a posterior acoustic shadow. **PRESENTATION:** • With reflective tissues, the posterior acoustic shadow is due to the almost total ultrasounds reflection. Since they cannot propagate in underlying tissues, that region does not yield any image. • Often, in these materials the posterior acoustic shadow is added to the reverberation artefact created by ultrasounds reflection, thus generating a dirty posterior acoustic shadow (Fig. 3.6). • With strongly attenuating tissues, most ultrasounds are absorbed, so they do not come back to the probe; again, lacking reflected echoes, there is no information about the underlying area. This generates a clean posterior acoustic shadow, i.e. fully anechoic (Fig. 3.7). **HOW TO REDUCE/PREVENT THEM:** • This artefact cannot be avoided or reduced, but must be used to differentiate normal intestinal ingesta from foreign bodies.
Mirror effect (Fig. 3.8)	**CAUSE:** • It is a form of reverberation caused by highly reflective curved interfaces, whose diameter is greater than the width of the ultrasound beam. • The mirror effect is often generated by the diaphragmatic–pleural interface. • Usually, ultrasounds leave the probe and meet the gallbladder that reflect them back to the probe. Some ultrasounds do not meet the gallbladder but rather the diaphragmatic interface; they are partly reflected towards the probe (creating the diaphragm image), and partly in a different direction. If these reflected echoes meet the gallbladder, they are reflected back again toward the diaphragmatic interface and from here to the probe (Fig. 3.8a). • The delay of these ultrasounds, compared to those that came back directly to the probe, indicates their deeper origin. **PRESENTATION:** • The mirror effect duplicates the image of a structure and place the artificial image in specular way compared to the surface that created the artefact (Fig. 3.8b). **HOW TO REDUCE/PREVENT THEM:** • The mirror effect cannot be avoided, but if a good mirror effect is lacking at the diaphragmatic interface, a thoracic pathology must be suspected.
Refraction or lateral acoustic shadows (Fig. 3.9)	**CAUSE:** • When the ultrasound beam hits the edge of a curved structure, ultrasounds are refracted; in other words, they change direction. • There are no return echoes from these edges, because echoes are no longer perpendicular to the angle of incidence, so do not hit the probe surface. **PRESENTATION:** • A posterior acoustic shadow is created at the point of maximum curvature due to lacking reflected echoes (Fig. 3.9). • Typical locations are kidneys, gallbladder, portal vessels and bladder. **HOW TO REDUCE/PREVENT THEM:** • They cannot be avoided, but must be recognized to avoid mistakes, as they can mime ruptures of bladder, gallbladder, etc.

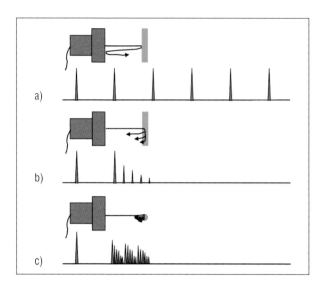

Figure 3.3 **a)** Repetition artefact: a smooth and regular surface reflects all the ultrasound beam simultaneously and this beam is uniformly reflected at probe level. Reflection intervals are generated that are regular and multiples of the distance between the two highly reflective structures. **b)** If the surface that creates the repetition artefact is not regular, additional hyperechoic echoes are generated that are not multiples of the distance between the two structures. This is the reverberation. **c)** If structures are very small, echoes are so close together to seem almost merged. This is the comet tail artefact.

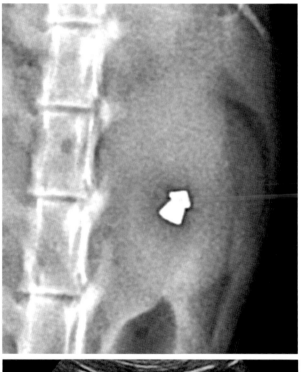

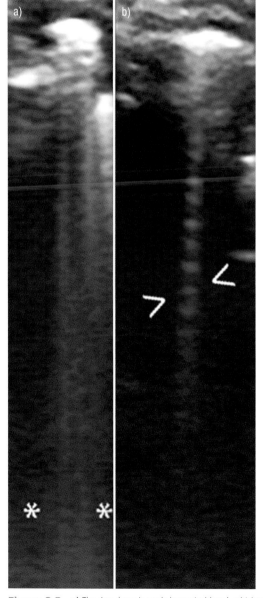

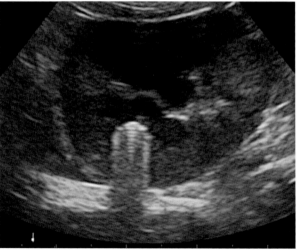

Figure 3.4 Reverberation artefact and "comet tail" created by a small metal body (bullet). You can differentiate it from a gas reverberation because here artefacts appear fixed, immobile, even.

Figure 3.5 **a)** The ring-down is made by vertical 'rays', which tend to expand and be more substantial with increasing depth (* *). **b)** The comet tail (> <) is identified observing the short parallel horizontal lines, which attenuate with depth.

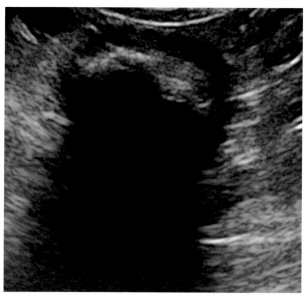

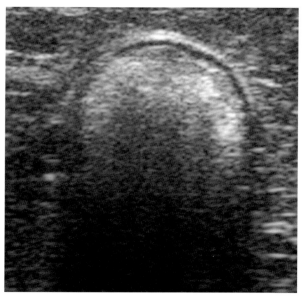

Figure 3.6 The colon in a patient. The mixed content of fecal material and gas creates a 'dirty' posterior shadowing, i.e. with different foci and echoic lines created by reverberation artefacts.

Figure 3.7 Foreign body in a small-intestine loop: a structure with thin hyperechoic interface associated to clean posterior shadowing (fully anechoic).

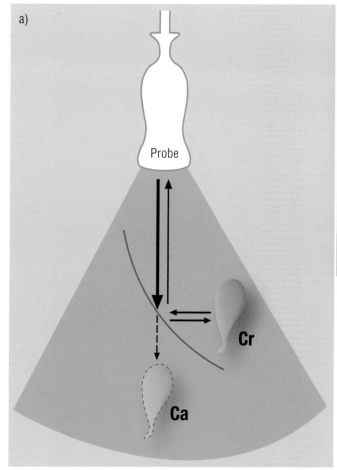

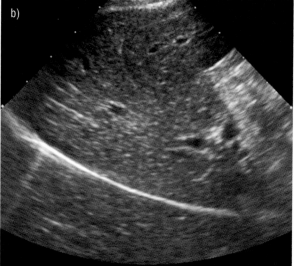

Figure 3.8 **a)** Mirror effect: rGa = real gallbladder; Ga = gallbladder created by the mirror effect. Some ultrasounds are reflected by the diaphragmatic interface toward the gallbladder, which acts as reflective interface and throws back part of these echoes to the diaphragmatic interface (the gradually thinner arrows show echoes that fade away). The computer postulates that the ultrasound beam has a straight path, and since echoes from the adventitious image reach the probe later compared to echoes coming from the interface they rose from, the ghost image is deeper than the diaphragm, in a specular way. **b)** Mirror effect at the diaphragmatic interface: the liver specular image is visualized in the chest. Note the small comet tail on the left of the image.

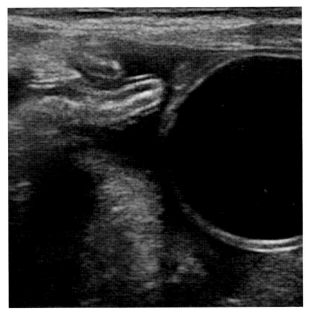

Figure 3.9 The bladder of this patient has a parietal gap in its most cranial portion, just at the curvature apex. Below the discontinuous curvature a shadowing is glimpsed. This parietal gap is an artefact created by deviation of ultrasounds when they meet a curved surface.

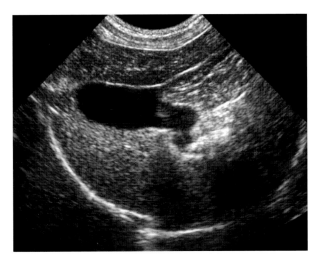

Figure 3.10 In the more superficial centimetre, note the uniformly echoic and coarsely textured band: this is the near-field artefact. There are no structures more superficial than the falciform ligament. This image shows also an artefact resulting from propagation speed error: the caudal portion of the gallbladder and the diaphragmatic interface to the left of the image appear broken off and placed deeper than their cranial portions. This step is due to the slowing of the ultrasound beam when it goes through the thick adipose layer of the falciform ligament, placed proximally to the caudal portion of the gallbladder. Taken from Spattini G: Gli artefatti in ecografia veterinaria: come riconoscerli e correggerli. Veterinaria, 22 (1): 9–20, 2008.

OBSERVED ARTEFACTS

Artefacts generated by the ultrasonographic device **Near-field artefact (Fig. 3.10)**	**CAUSE:** • The probe contains piezoelectric crystals which convert electrical impulses into ultrasounds and vice versa. • Crystals include several vibrating points that interact together and create a wavefront that saturates the image, not allowing for the real representation of the patient tissues in the first few millimetres in contact with the probe. **PRESENTATION:** • All ultrasonographic images show this artefact. • The near-field artefact thickness also decreases when the probe frequency increases (Fig. 3.10). Linear probes have the smallest artefact thickness. **HOW TO REDUCE/PREVENT THEM:** • The near-field artefact cannot be avoided, so the region of interest must not fall in the near-field artefact area; common examples are the superficial portion of the feline spleen and the bladder ventral wall. • To create diagnostic images from these very superficial structures, silicon spacers or even latex gloves filled with water can be used, taking care to not leave air bubbles inside. Moreover, multiple scan planes can be used to be sure that images are obtained from all portions of target organs, without the need for spacers.
Propagation speed error artefact (Fig. 3.10).	**CAUSE:** • The computer postulates the ultrasounds speed in tissues is constant. This way, the more time elapses between the ultrasound emission and the return of its echo to the probe, the greater the distance where reflection happened. • If the propagation speed is constant, the ultrasound that comes back first will have covered a lesser distance than the ultrasound that comes back later. • Actually, speed of ultrasounds in soft tissues is similar but not constant. • The adipose tissue has the greatest variation with 1480 m/s versus 1540 m/s of other tissues. **PRESENTATION:** • The difference in propagation speed falsely changes the depth of structures that are behind a layer of adipose tissue, putting them on a deeper level compared to the real one (Fig. 3.10).

OBSERVED ARTEFACTS (Continued)

Propagation speed error artefact (Fig. 3.10).	**HOW TO REDUCE/PREVENT THEM:** • This artefact cannot be avoided, but must be recognized so as to not think the diaphragmatic interface or the gallbladder are broken up, thus damaged. • Scan angles can be changed to avoid different layers of adipose tissue appearing superficial compared to the evaluated structure.
Posterior-wall enhancement (Fig. 3.11).	**CAUSE:** • The computer postulates that the ultrasound beam propagates in tissues at constant speed and attenuates in a uniform and proportional way compared to the length of crossed-through path. • Following these postulates, the computer concludes that reflected echoes that come back first to the probe have travelled less and are less attenuated, while ultrasounds that come back later to the probe have travelled more and are more attenuated. • To counterbalance the attenuation effect and produce uniform images, the computer reduces the echogenicity of more superficial echoes and amplifies those of deep echoes. • However, ultrasounds crossing fluid collections are less attenuated compared to those travelling in soft tissues. **PRESENTATION:** • Tissues that are distal to fluid collections appear uniformly hyperechoic compared to surrounding tissues (Fig. 3.11). • This artefact occurs if the density of crossed tissue is lower than soft tissues; so, it may be that this artefact is absent distally to an abscess whose density, despite its 'fluid' content, is close to parenchymal organs. **HOW TO REDUCE/PREVENT THEM:** • The posterior-wall enhancement artefact cannot be avoided. • Such artefact is considered pathognomonic of a fluid collection and is useful in differentiating an anechoic nodule from a cyst: if the material is anechoic but parenchymal, there will be no posterior-wall enhancement. • A second way to differentiate a nodule from a cyst is maximizing the gain: if the structure is a cyst, the difference in echogenicity between cyst and surrounding tissues will be greater; on the contrary, if the structure is an anechoic parenchyma, i.e. contains material able to generate echoes, the difference in echogenicity will be lower.
Partial-volume artefact	**CAUSE:** • The ultrasound beam is three-dimensional and features height, width and thickness. • It can be imagined as a piece of cake. The computer creates a two-dimensional image starting from three-dimensional data, and averaging data obtained from the thickness. • Echoic and anechoic structures are added together, and intermediate echogenicities are inserted into the image: this creates the partial-volume artefact. **PRESENTATION:** • •When images are obtained from the peripheral bladder, the primary beam can collect information regarding both the bladder wall and the urine, producing a 'pseudo-sediment' image. **HOW TO REDUCE/PREVENT THEM:** • There are several ways to differentiate a genuine sediment from a 'pseudo-sediment'. The surface of the 'pseudo-sediment' is curved, while the surface of the genuine sediment is flat. • Just tilting the probe slightly and moving more toward the centre of the bladder removes the artefact. When in doubt, the patient recumbency can be changed to see if sediment shape and position change.
Partial-volume artefact	• The 'pseudo-sediment' is more marked in the focal region where the thickness of the ultrasound beam is electronically compressed and the mean calculated over more data. If the image focus is moved, the artefact can be reduced. Actually, all ultrasonographic images contain the partial-volume artefact but this is only visible with anechoic structures.
Side-lobe artefact (Fig. 3.12–13)	**CAUSE:** • The computer postulates that the probe emits a single ultrasound beam at right angles to the probe surface. • Actually, there are secondary beams at opposite ends of the primary beam. • These beams are created by piezoelectric crystals, have different directions compared to the primary beam, and have a lower intensity.

OBSERVED ARTEFACTS (Continued)

Side-lobe artefact (Fig. 3.12–13)	• They do not create visible effects within an echoic image, but if a significant amount of the image is anechoic, weak echoes of side beams are visible. • The computer postulates that all echoes arise from the primary beam, so echoes from secondary side beams are shown in the centre of the image, as if they were raised from the main beam (Fig. 3.12). **PRESENTATION:** • This artefact concurs to form the bladder 'pseudo-sediment', together with the partial-volume artefact, but unlike the pseudo-sediment, the surface is not curved. • Bladder, gallbladder and large collections of anechoic fluids are the locations where the artefact is more often found. • For example, the colon adjoining the bladder can create weak echoes that appear within the bladder (Fig. 3.13). **HOW TO REDUCE/PREVENT THEM:** • Usually, to reduce side-lobe artefacts, simply decreasing the overall gain is needed, so removing low-energy echoes; this way, artefacts can be nearly eradicated without reducing the image detail.

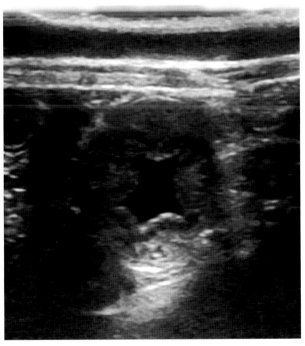

Figure 3.11   Foetal resorption. Note that tissues below the anechoic collection are hyperechoic compared to surrounding tissues. This is the posterior-wall enhancement effect.

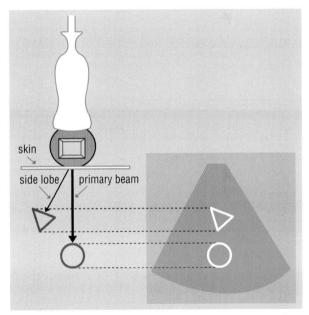

Figure 3.12   a) One side beam sends and receives reflected echoes from a structure located along its path (triangle). The computer ignores lateral beams and postulates that all reflected echoes are generated by the main ultrasound beam that propagates axially (circle). So, structures that are not hit by the primary beam, but by lateral beams, are erroneously shown as if they were on the same axis of the main beam; in other words, they are shown in a fake place. **b)** In the final image, the triangle is at the right depth but on the wrong plane.

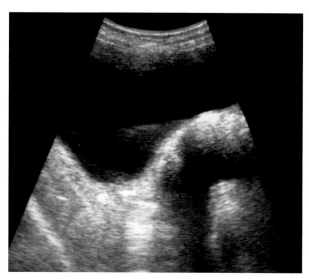

Figure 3.13 Due to 'side lobes', echoes generated by the colon are visualized within the bladder. Taken from Spattini G: Gli artefatti in ecografia veterinaria: come riconoscerli e correggerli. Veterinaria, 22(1): 9–20, 2008.

RECOMMENDED READING

Louvet A, Bourgeois JM: Lung ring down artifact as a sign of pulmonary alveolar-interstitial disease. Vet Radiol & Ultrasound. 2008, 49(4): 374–377.

Reef VB: Artifacts. In: Reef VB: Equine diagnostic ultrasound. WB Saunders Co. 1998, pp: 24–38.

Kirberger RM: Imaging artifacts in diagnostic ultrasound—A review. Vet Rad & Ultrasound. 1995, 36: 297–306.

Ziskin MC, Tickman DI, Goldenberg NJ, Lapayowker MS, Becker JM. The comet tail artifact. J Ultrasound Med. 1982, 1: 1–7.

4

Scan technique in ultrasonography and ultrasonographic landmarks

Federica Rossi

PATIENT PREPARATION

To make the abdominal ultrasonographic examination easier the following measures are to be adopted.

Abstinence from food	• 12 hours at least: a highly-distended stomach prevents the proper assessment of left cranial abdomen; moreover, if there is some food, the gastric wall is difficult to assess. Emergency situations are clearly the only exception.
Carminative drugs	• They are not effective in small animals so are not recommended.
Water	• When administered orally (15 ml/kg), it can be useful to relax the stomach if the gastric wall is to be evaluated.
Fecal content in large intestine	• If abundant, it can hinder the ultrasonographic examination, so the owner must be advised to let the animal defecate before the exam.
Bladder repletion	• To evaluate the urinary tract to the smallest details, it is important that the bladder is stretched. The wall of an empty bladder is falsely thickened, so the organ cannot be evaluated.
Sedation	• It is essential if the patient is not cooperative. The environment must be quiet, noiseless and in half-light, to easily visualize images on the monitor.

PREPARATION OF AREA TO BE EXAMINED

Hair-clipping	• Abdomen: it must include an area that comes from the xyphoid process to the pubic region, reaching laterally the last two intercostal spaces (evaluation of hepatic lobes) and flanks (evaluation of the retroperitoneal space). The hair-clipper must be used carefully, to avoid skin injuries. • Chest and neck: it depends on the area of interest.
Alcohol	• It is useful to remove hair remnants, skin debris, and the air they withhold. • Do not apply alcohol to skin injuries, nor directly on the probe.
Gel	• It is essential to obtain optimal contact between probe and skin; it must be applied plentifully and repeatedly even during the exam. Note that it must be removed before fine-needle aspirates, otherwise the gel will pollute the sample.

PATIENT POSITIONING

The patient positioning must be convenient for the operator, comfortable and relaxing for the patient, and must allow for undisturbed examination by the ultrasonographer.

Mattress	• A soft mattress facilitates the examination, as the animal is more comfortable and better tolerates the procedure.
Restraint	• The animal must be immobile: a gentle restraint is required, with the support of one or two helpers. In most cases one person is enough, notably adopting the lateral recumbency.
Recumbency: the abdomen	• The recumbency must be changed, if needed. In most cases, start with a standard recumbency (right lateral or dorsal), then move the animal in another recumbency, if needed. • The advantage of dorsal recumbency (Fig. 4.1a) is that it equally exposes both hemiabdomens and allows for a symmetrical positioning that is more close to a surgical approach. Nevertheless, it is less comfortable for the animal, even using a positioning cushion. • The advantage of right lateral recumbency (Fig. 4.1b) is to be more comfortable and more tolerated by the animal. It provides an excellent window to the left caudal, middle, and cranial abdomen. To explore the right cranial abdomen, the hand and probe must be placed between the abdominal wall and the table (Fig. 4.2). This may be quite difficult, but there is a considerable practical advantage: the gas tends to shift dorsally moving away from these regions; therefore, the study of organs such as the pyloric region of the stomach, the duodenum and the pancreas is facilitated. With this recumbency, notably in large breed dogs, it is not always possible to properly examine the kidney and the right adrenal gland, so the animal must be moved in dorsal recumbency or left lateral recumbency. • The left lateral recumbency can be useful to examine right side organs (for example, an intercostal scan for right liver lobes). • The exam of a dog in quadrupedal posture is not optimal for a careful abdominal study as the patient may still move; so, accurate standard scans from the various organs are very difficult to obtain. This position can be used to evaluate special situations (e.g. animals with severe dyspnoea) and investigate certain organs or injuries exploiting the gravity effect to the end of a conventional examination (for example, bladder stones or gastric foreign bodies).
Recumbency: the thorax	• The patient's clinical status must be always considered; in case of severe dyspnoea (for example, a subject with pleural effusion) the sternal recumbency or the quadrupedal posture is preferable. • The recumbency (Fig. 4.3a) must be selected according to the injury site; moreover, a pleural effusion may facilitate the visualization of injuries, so that effusion can be 'moved' as needed. • Sometimes, leaving the patient in lateral recumbency for a few minutes makes a lung injury easier to visualize, because the dependent lung develops atelectasis and the injury comes in contact with the thoracic wall. In this case, a procedure table with openings is useful to perform a scan in a ventral position.
Recumbency: the neck	• The ventral neck region can be examined using the sternal recumbency or the quadrupedal posture (Fig. 4.3b). If the animal is calm and collaborative, this is the most physiological condition and allows one to evaluate larynx movements as well. • However, the dorsal recumbency is often needed, restraining the subject with its head extended in a symmetrical way: this is the only way to properly evaluate regional small structures (thyroid lobes, lymph nodes, salivary glands).

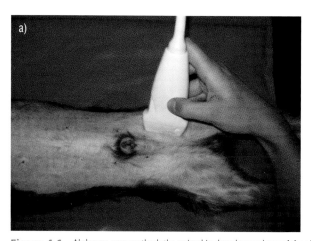

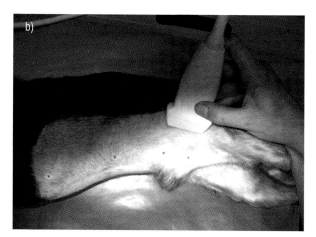

Figure 4.1 Abdomen scan method: the animal in dorsal recumbency **(a)** or lateral recumbency **(b)**. Note the broad hair-clipping, also including last intercostal spaces.

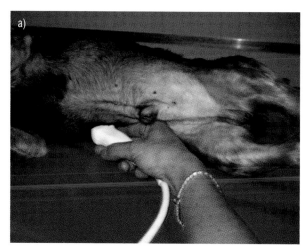

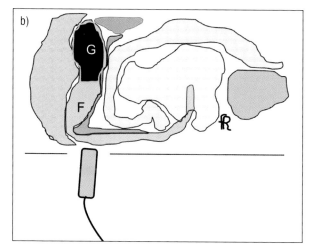

Figure 4.2 The picture **(a)** shows how to scan the right cranial abdomen with the animal in right lateral recumbency. The diagram **(b)** demonstrates the usefulness of this positioning to scan the gastric antrum and proximal duodenum, where fluid (F) accumulates, and the right pancreatic lobe. With this position, the gas (G) moves in the gastric fundus region.

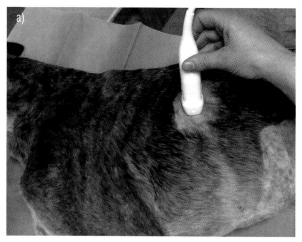

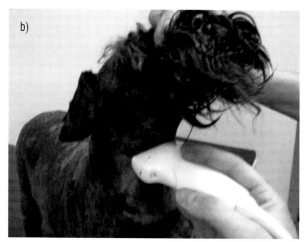

Figure 4.3 Scan method for the chest with the animal in lateral recumbency **(a)** and for the ventral neck in quadrupedal posture **(b)**.

ARRANGEMENT AND OPERATOR DEXTERITY

Patient, operator and equipment arrangement	• The most used arrangement is the table to the right, the operator sitting at the left and facing the ultrasonographic device. The table and chair height must provide a comfortable position to the arms, especially if the ultrasonographic device must be operated for several hours. A height-adjustable table may be useful, possibly with an opening which can be used to scan from beneath, or to add an echocardiography.
Hands	• The right hand is used to move the probe, while the left hand operates the machine.
Left-handed operators	• Most left-handed ultrasonographers (and some are renowned!!!) prefer using the same arrangement of right-handed operators. So, manual ability to move the probe on the patient with the non-dominant hand must be acquired, and this may be more difficult. However, using the specular arrangement, understanding and acquiring standard positions (for example, those indicated on textbooks and used by most operators) is more difficult.
Dexterity during procedures (FNA, biopsies)	• For right-handed ultrasonographers, the author suggests reversing your hands during procedures. Once the target injury or organ is identified, change the hand and keep the probe still with your left hand, which is not difficult since the probe must stay immobile. The right hand (dominant) is then used to insert tools (needles or catheters). For left-handed operators, reversing hands is not needed. During procedures, a helper is always wise.

PROBE MOVEMENTS (Fig. 4.4–7)

During the ultrasonographic examination, different movements are needed, which combined together make it possible to thoroughly examine a structure or organ:

- Translation (Fig. 4.4)
- Tilting (Fig. 4.5)
- Rotation (Fig. 4.6)
- Rocking (Fig. 4.7)

Manual dexterity is acquired by gaining experience (for YEARS, not days or weeks!).

Once an organ or structure is identified, you must learn to make small adjustment movements, optimize the scan and make the image clearer and more diagnostic.

Keeping the same position for a bit is already a way to have a better image, as it improves the contact between probe and skin, optimally distributes the gel and moves the air entrapped in residual hair. With time, these movements become automatic, and are mixed using the teaching subdivision previously described.

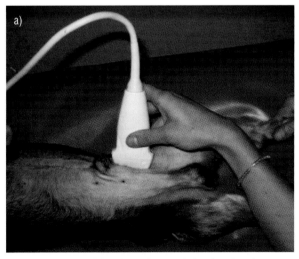
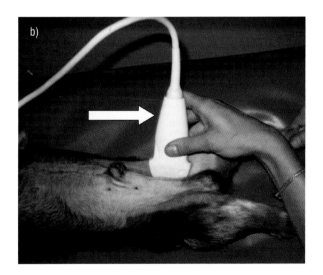

Figure 4.4 Probe sliding along a horizontal plane (translation).

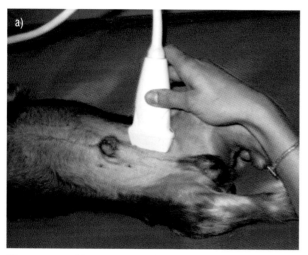
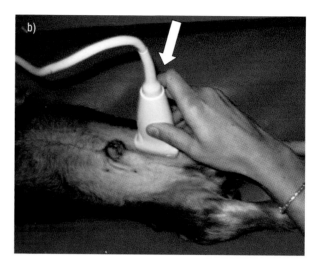

Figure 4.5 Obliquity movements (tilting).

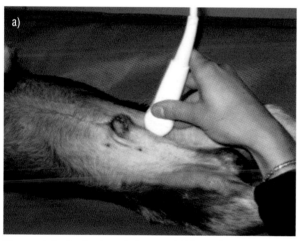
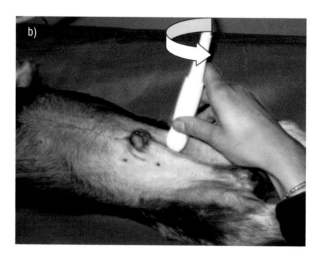

Figure 4.6 Turning the probe by an angle (often 90°) on its axis (rotation).

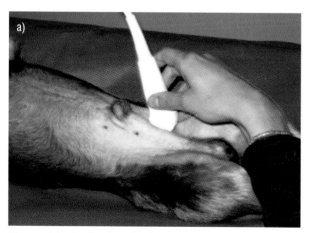
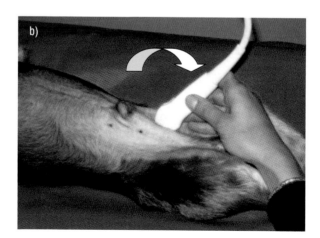

Figure 4.7 Bending the probe along its longitudinal axis (rocking).

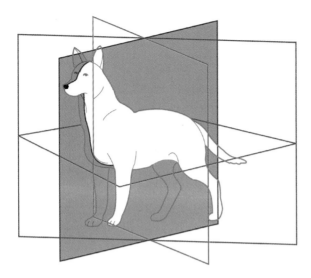

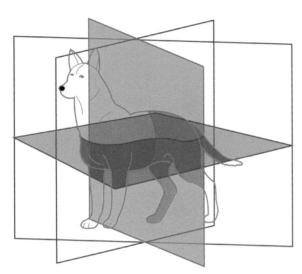

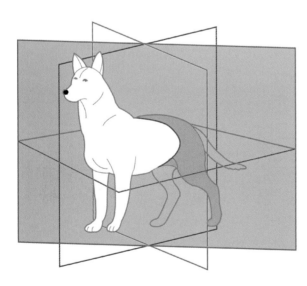

SCAN PLANES (Fig. 4.8)

Knowing and using various standard scan planes for various organs is important, so the normal image of a structure can be acquired; then, images can be compared with pathologic ones seen at training courses, in textbooks or journal articles.
Different standard scan planes (Fig. 4.8) are:

- Longitudinal
- Transverse
- Dorsal (coronal)
- Oblique.

ULTRASONOGRAPHIC IMAGE ORIENTATION (Fig. 4.9–12)

- Ultrasonographic images must be oriented to comply with certain rules shared throughout the scientific world.
- By convention:
  - For images obtained in the longitudinal scan (Fig. 4.9), the image on the left side indicates the cranial side of the animal/organ, while the right side indicates the caudal side;
  - For images obtained in the transverse scan (Fig. 4.10), the image on the left side indicates the right side of the animal/organ, while the right side indicates the left side.
- For a correct orientation, you must check how the probe is positioned over the animal. Each probe has a marker indicating one of its sides.
- The marker is matched with the monitor of the ultrasonographic device, and indicated by a symbol that can be on the right or left side of the ultrasonographic image.
- The marker on the probe, and the symbol on the monitor, must match so there is always a proper correspondence between the animal side and the ultrasonographic image side; in other words:
  - If the marker is oriented towards the cranial portion (longitudinal scan, Fig. 4.9) or to the right of the animal (transverse scan, Fig. 4.10), in the image, the marker must appear to the left side of the monitor;
  - If the marker is oriented towards the caudal portion (longitudinal scan, Fig. 4.11) or to the left of the animal (transverse scan, Fig. 4.12), in the image, the marker must appear to the right side of the monitor;
  - To switch from the longitudinal scan to the transverse scan, the probe must be rotated by 90 degrees counter-clockwise.

LONGITUDINAL SCAN PLANE
DORSAL SCAN PLANE
OBLIQUE SCAN PLANE

Figure 4.8 Standard scan planes.

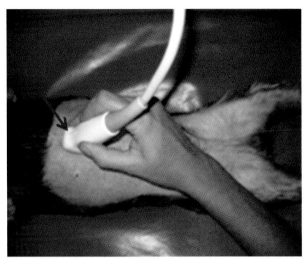

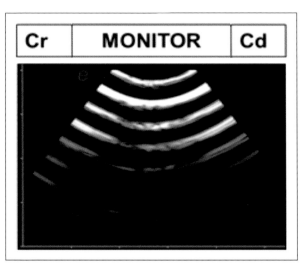

Figure 4.9   Longitudinal scan. The marker (red arrow) is aligned towards the cranial part of the animal and to the left in the image ('e' symbol).

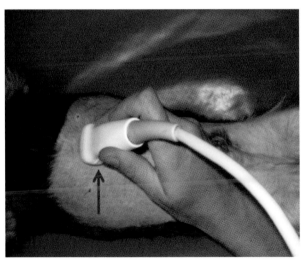

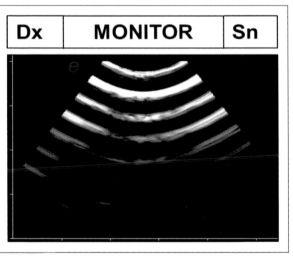

Figure 4.10   Transverse scan. The marker (red arrow) is aligned towards the right part of the animal and to the left in the image ('e' symbol). The probe is rotated by 90° counter-clockwise, compared to the previous image.

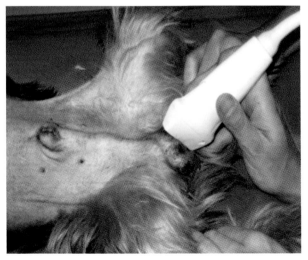

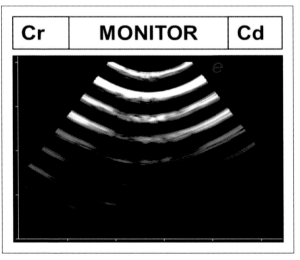

Figure 4.11   Longitudinal scan. The marker (red arrow) is aligned towards the caudal part of the animal and to the right in the image ('e' symbol).

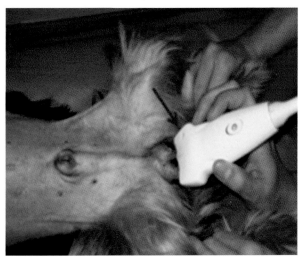

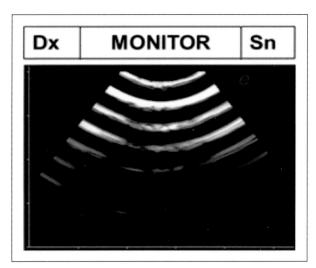

Figure 4.12 Transverse scan. The marker (red arrow) is aligned towards the left part of the animal and to the right in the image ('e' symbol). The probe is rotated by 90° counter-clockwise, compared to the previous image.

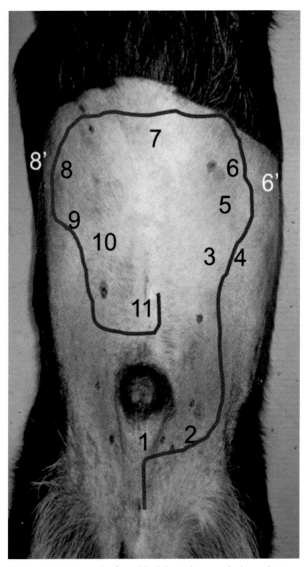

Figure 4.13 Example of possible abdominal scan-method according to positions from 1 to 11. In the end, from position 11, the probe can be moved laterally to the right flank, then moved caudally to identify the bladder again.

PERFORMING THE ULTRASONOGRAPHIC EXAMINATION (Fig. 4.13)

Learning how to perform the ultrasonographic examination following a systematic approach is extremely important. This means:

- To identify all structures/organs visible on ultrasonography
- To investigate each of them, through all scan planes
- Do not be swayed by obvious injuries or lesions suspected according to the clinical examination

To establish a personal method to perform a full examination. The order and sequence of examined organs may vary, but repeating movements always in the same way helps to learn the technique without missing one or more structures.

Figure 4.13 shows one of possible scan methods, useful to focus the different basic positions (numbered from 1 to 11) to find the abdominal structures to be examined. The animal is in right lateral recumbency, or in dorsal recumbency. The probe is moved from position 1 to 11 following a kind of question mark, beginning at the caudal abdomen, continuing cranially on the abdomen left side, then ending at the middle and right cranial part. Remaining on the right side, go caudally along the abdominal wall, and finish examining the central abdominal region.

A series of diagrams is shown with relationships between positions shown in Fig. 4.13 and main abdominal anatomical structures.

Diagram 14 shows main organs of gastrointestinal and urinary systems.

Diagram 15 shows locations of main abdominal lymphocentres compared to the reproductive system.

Table 4.1 summarizes the main structures found in each position indicated in Fig. 4.13, and some useful landmarks. In each chapter, the table dedicated to the scan technique shows more details and tips for finding abdominal organs.

a)

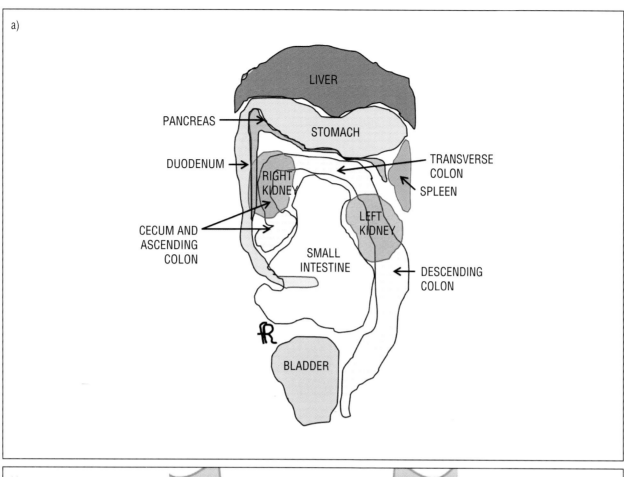

b)

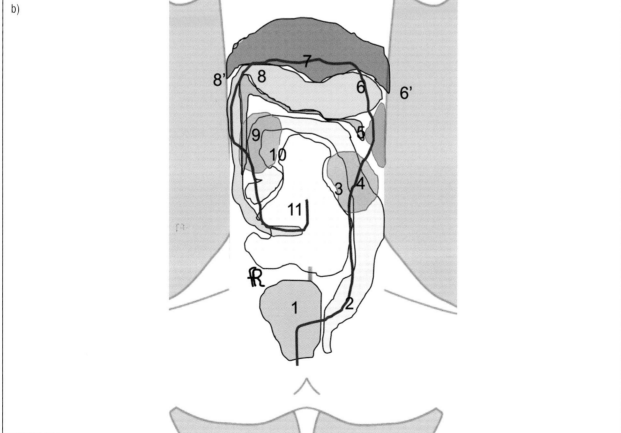

Figure 4.14 Diagrams representing various abdominal organs in the ventral view **(a)**, and relationships with different scan positions **(b)**.

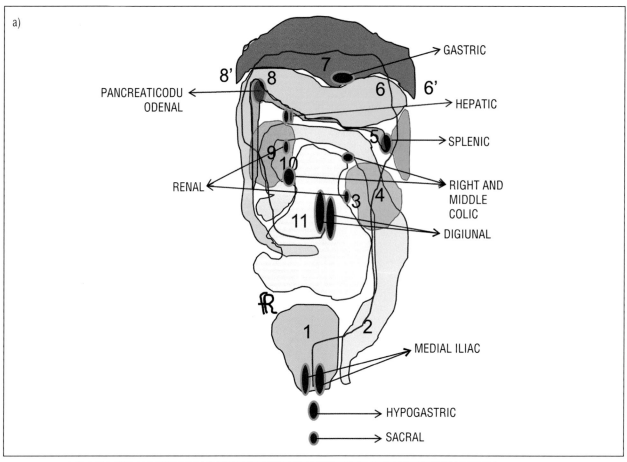

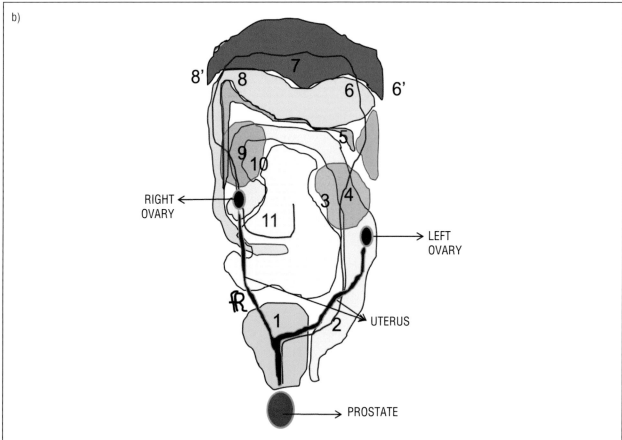

Figure 4.15   Diagrams representing the location of main groups of abdominal lymph nodes **(a)** and the reproductive system **(b)**.

Table 4.1
Main organs/structures found in positions from 1 to 11 (Fig. 4.13) and ultrasound landmarks

Position	Probe	Visible organs	Scans	Comments
1	Caudal abdomen, cranially to the pubis, mid-line	Bladder, colon, prostate, corpus uteri	Longitudinal and transverse	
2	Caudal abdomen, on the left of mid-line, the probe is slightly ventrally to lumbar rachis	Vessels (aorta and iliac arteries, caudal vena cava and iliac veins), iliac lymph nodes	Longitudinal and transverse	The Doppler is useful to identify vessels and obtain blood flows
From 2 to 3	Caudal abdomen, on the left of mid-line, the probe is slightly ventrally to lumbar rachis	Aorta and caudal vena cava, lymph nodes when enlarged; renal vessels and left adrenal gland sometimes visible	Longitudinal and transverse	Arteries going out from the aorta (renal artery, cranial mesenteric and celiac arteries) are the landmarks to identify the left adrenal gland
4	Middle abdomen on the left, slightly lateral to the previous scan	Left kidney, left ovary	Longitudinal, transverse and dorsal	For the kidney dorsal scan, moving the probe in one of the last intercostal spaces is sometimes needed
5	Cranial abdomen, on the left	Spleen, small intestine, transverse and descending colon, pancreas left lobe	Longitudinal, transverse and oblique	The splenic head position is fixed; then, continue towards the middle abdomen, following variable contours of splenic body and splenic tail
6	Cranial abdomen, on the left, in contact with the costal arch	Stomach (fundus), left hepatic lobes	Longitudinal, transverse and oblique	The visualization of hepatic lobes varies depending on the gastric filling and content
6'	Left intercostal scan	Left liver lobes	As allowed by the intercostal space	
7	Mid-line, the probe in contact with the xyphoid process	Liver (cranially oriented probe), stomach and pancreas bodies (more perpendicularly oriented probe)	Longitudinal and transverse	Excellent liver overview
8	Cranial abdomen, on the right, in contact with the costal arch	Liver (right lobes), porta hepatis (vessels), gallbladder and common bile duct, stomach (pylorus), duodenum, pancreas (body and right lobe)	Longitudinal, transverse and oblique	For this scan the right lateral recumbency is useful (gas is removed from stomach and duodenum); see Fig. 4.2
8'	Right intercostal scan	Right liver lobes	As allowed by the intercostal space	Directing the probe caudoventrally an oblique scan is obtained that shows the three main abdominal vessels (aorta, caudal vena cava and portal vein); this is useful when suspecting a vascular anomaly
9	Middle abdomen, to the right	Right kidney, duodenum, pancreas (right lobe), right ovary	Longitudinal, transverse and dorsal	For the kidney dorsal scan, moving the probe in one of last intercostal spaces is sometimes needed
10	Middle abdomen, to the right, slightly medially compared to the previous scan	Caudal vena cava and right adrenal gland	Longitudinal and transverse	Landmark to find the right adrenal gland: the caudal vena cava
11	Middle abdomen, central position	Small intestine, jejunal and colic lymph nodes, peritoneum, ascending and transverse colon	Longitudinal, transverse and oblique	Mesenteric vessels: the landmark for jejunal lymph nodes

5 Interventional techniques in ultrasonography

Federica Rossi

INDICATIONS

Several interventional procedures are currently used in veterinary medicine for the purpose of:

- Getting the diagnosis of a disease, and among others:
  - collection of fluid samples from cavities (cytological examination and culture), e.g. cystocentesis, pyelocentesis, thoracentesis, cholecystocentesis;
  - needle aspirate from cystic or solid injuries. FNA (Fine Needle Aspiration) is an aspiration performed with a <20 G needle; these samples are used for the cytological examination;
  - cutting-needle biopsy (Tissue Core Biopsy, TCB) for solid masses. A tissue frustule is acquired and used for the histological examination;
  - injection of contrast agent in a cavity to perform radiographic studies: e.g. descending ureterography.
- Aid to treat injuries:
  - positioning of catheters/drainages
  - alcoholization of cysts/abscesses
  - ablation with radiofrequencies/microwaves
  - intraoperative procedures.

There are basically two BENEFITS from using the ultrasonographic assistance compared with other methods (blind biopsy or fluoroscopic/tomographic biopsy):

- The direct real-time visualization of the needle during the procedure increases its success and safety.
- There is no exposure to ionizing radiation.

FNA AND TCB (Table 5.1)

PATIENT PREPARATION
- Before the cutting-needle biopsy of any structure, or the needle aspiration of well-vascularized organ or injury, make sure to rule out a coagulopathy that may increase the bleeding risk. Information coming from history and clinical examination must be combined with laboratory tests results (complete blood count and coagulation panel), which are always needed before any procedure.
- The needle aspiration is a quick and minimally invasive procedure; it is generally well tolerated by the animal, so can be performed with the animal awake, reserving sedation to particularly restless subjects. To do a biopsy, however, a deep sedation or anaesthesia is needed, as the procedure is more invasive and a patient's sudden movement could cause serious damage to the examined organ. The anaesthetic protocol must always include an analgesic drug.

- The needed steps include broad hair-clipping, skin cleansing and surgical disinfection of the skin and the ultrasonographic probe. To obtain the right contact between skin and probe, alcohol is used rather than gel. Actually, the gel can penetrate the needle and contaminate the sample.

INSTRUMENTS
It is important that all needed material is neatly arranged and ready-to-serve, to speed up and optimize the procedure. A cart equipped for that particular purpose is very useful.

1. An ultrasonographic equipment fitted with a probe (linear, convex, sectoral) whose frequency is tailored to the proper visualization of the injury.
   There are probes dedicated to biopsy procedures that have a slot to insert the needle into. An alternative to these probes are biopsy needle guides (Fig. 5.5b); they can be mounted on any normal probe and have a housing for the probe and a sliding channel for the needle. Dedicated probes and guides must be sterilized before use. Note that each type of probe needs a different guide. Using a guide can be avoided if the operator adopts the freehand technique.
2. Needles: 21-25 G hypodermic needles or 20-22 G spinal needles can be used; the latter have the advantage that the mandrel prevents collecting cells in the needle before reaching the injury. Long spinal needles may be useful to achieve deeper injuries, but they are sometimes difficult to direct.
3. Intravenous catheters: they are used by some ultrasonographers, e.g. for the needle aspiration of some highly vascular parenchymatous organs (e.g. the spleen).
4. To aspirate cavities or in alcoholization procedures, a set with syringe, three-way stopcock, extension and needle is very useful (Fig. 5.1).

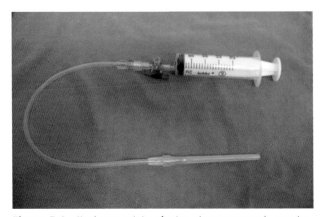

Figure 5.1 Simple set consisting of syringe, three-way stopcock, extension and needle. It is useful for procedures that require aspirating fluid collections and possibly injecting contrast agent, alcohol, or other material.

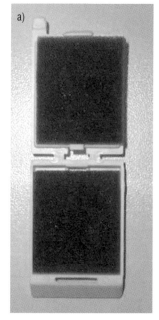
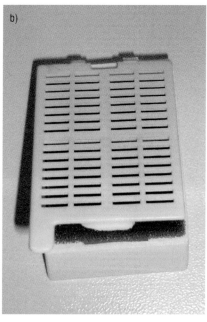

Figure 5.2 Embedding cassettes, open **(a)** and closed **(b)**, useful to contain and protect small biopsy specimens.

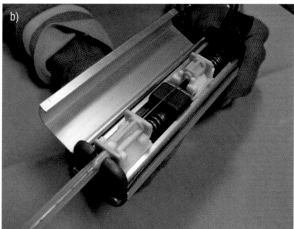

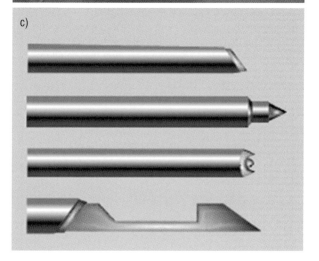

5. Material for disinfection.
6. Material for sample storage and transport; slides, embedding cassettes (Fig. 5.2), test tubes with formalin.
7. Instruments for TCB (Fig. 5.3). Several tools are useful, based on:
   – Cutting mechanism: manual, semi-automatic or automatic. Manual instruments are introduced and activated manually; the disadvantage is that both hands must be used, so help is needed during the procedure. Semi-automatic and automatic instruments can be operated with one hand and are the most used today. Semi-automatic instruments have a manual first step (introduction), while the second step is automatic (cutting); in contrast, automatic instruments have two automatic steps that follow each other rapidly.
   – Gauge: variable between 14 G and 20 G.
   – Type of shearing portion (Fig. 5.3).
   – Length of shearing portion: for most needles it is 1–2 cm and must be selected according to the injury size.

OPERATIVE TECHNIQUE (Tables 5.2 and 5.3)

The guiding principle for all these methods is that all procedural steps are mandatory.

To accomplish that, the used instrument (needle, catheter, etc.) must be included within the ultrasound beam during the whole procedure, according to the triangulation rule (Fig. 5.4).

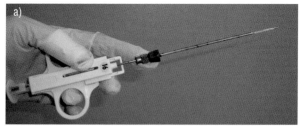

◀ **Figure 5.3** Semi-automatic **(a)** and automatic **(b)** biopsy needle; **c)** Different types of shearing portion.

TABLE 5.1 How to choose between FNA and TCB	
The following points are to be considered:	
The patient and its general health state	• Lab tests (blood count and coagulation panel); if values are changed, avoid the TCB. • Deep sedation or anaesthesia abilities: if impossible, opt for FNA.
Type of injury to sample	Consider chances of getting a reliable diagnosis with the used method. As for cytological examination, chances of having a diagnostic result depend on the tendency of injury to yield cellular material. For example, with a clinical suspicion of lymphoma or mast cell tumour, the cytology likely leads to a diagnosis, so starting with FNA is recommended. On the other hand, with a renal or hepatic diffuse injury, the diagnosis requires evaluating the organ parenchyma architecture, so a TCB is needed.
Injury size	If less than about 1 cm, opt for FNA; if more than 1–2 cm, chose either FNA or TCB.
Injury vascularization (using Doppler)	If the injury has very huge vascular component, bleeding during TCB is much more likely, so opt for FNA.
Personal preference	Each operator must also choose according to their dexterity and experience in performing these procedures.
General guidelines	The right choice is starting with the least invasive method that probably provides a diagnostic result. So, often, FNA is the first choice, followed by the TCB if the cytology result is not satisfactory.
	Even if a TCB is performed, making a series of slides is recommended; they are enclosed with the biopsy sample and are sometimes useful for the diagnosis.

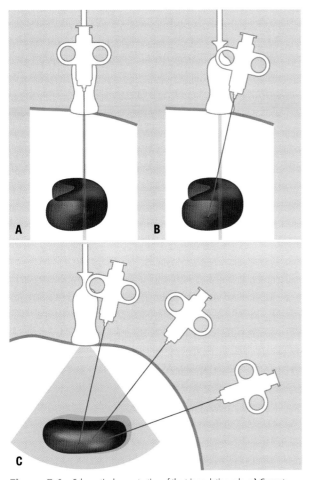

Figure 5.4 Schematic demonstration of the triangulation rule. **a)** Correct position of the needle, all aligned with the ultrasound beam. **b)** Wrong position; only a portion of the needle is included within the ultrasound beam, so is visualized, but control on the most important part of the needle (the tip) is lost. **c)** In all three positions the needle tip is correctly visualized. Depending on the selected introduction angle, a different needle portion is visualized. If the needle is close to the probe, the portion is longer, and this makes the procedure easier and safer.

ULTRASONOGRAPHIC ASSISTANCE OR FREEHAND (Fig. 5.5)

FNA or TCB can be performed using the ultrasonographic guidance or the freehand technique. Table 5.2 shows advantages and disadvantages for the two different techniques.

FNA TECHNIQUE

- Re-check the injury location
- Identify the shortest and safest path. Try to get as close as possible to the injury, without interposing any organs between the skin and the target point. Don't cross more than one cavity or organ.
- Introduce the needle quickly and control its position until it penetrates the injury (Fig. 5.6).
- There are two different techniques:
  - Needle aspiration: do a back and forth motion with the plunger without moving the syringe. Stop the suction before drawing the needle.
  - Needle puncture: drive the needle in the injury without aspirating; this is especially useful with highly vascular injuries as there is no blood aspiration that could reduce the method accuracy.
- To increase the method success, take at least three samples from each injury.
- Discard preparations with high blood content.
- Recheck the subject before discharge.

TCB TECHNIQUE

- Re-check the injury location by measuring the path the needle must follow to reach it.
- Use the Doppler to visualize large vessels you must avoid.

TABLE 5.2 Sampling techniques with ultrasonographic guidance or freehand technique: advantages and disadvantages

	Advantages	Disadvantages
ULTRASONOGRAPHIC GUIDANCE*	The needle tip is automatically included in the probe scan plane, so particular training in triangulation is not needed.	The needle is in contact with the needle-guide, so the latter must be sterile as well. Even the probe must be covered with a sterile glove or a probe cover.
		The angle between the ultrasound beam and the probe is fixed and this allows for less flexibility. This can be a problem if the injury is too shallow or too deep.
		The needle-guide kit, its sterilization and the sterile material are expensive.
		Each type of probe needs a different needle-guide kit.
FREEHAND TECHNIQUE*	Greater flexibility in reaching all injury types and sampling different parts of injury.	More experience needed.
	Fast procedure if the operator is experienced.	If the operator is inexperienced: more time to find the correct alignment between the needle and the probe.
	Less expensive material.	

* The literature reports the same diagnostic accuracy for the same operator experience.

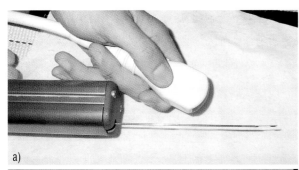

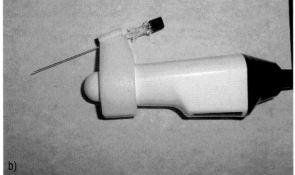

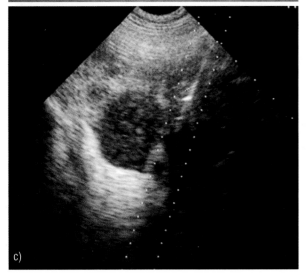

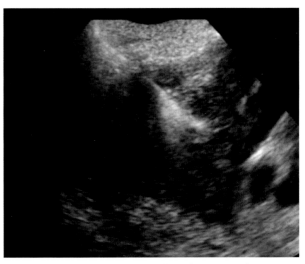

Figure 5.6 Ultrasonographic image obtained during FNA of a cat mediastinal mass. The needle is visible as a hyperechoic line that deepens in the injury until it reaches the centre.

- If the animal is only sedated, an injectable local anaesthetic at the needle puncture point is recommended.
- Make a small incision on the skin with a scalpel blade.
- Advance the needle until the proximal portion of the injury, then press the plunger (Fig. 5.7).
- Sample from several parts of the injury.
- Immediately after sampling, then at regular intervals, recheck the animal to detect any signs of haemorrhage

◀ **Figure 5.5 a)** Freehand biopsy: the triangulation between ultrasound beam and needle must be obtained manually. **b)** Ultrasonographic guidance: the needle is automatically included in the beam. **c)** Ultrasonographic image obtained under ultrasonographic assistance. Two dotted lines are visualized that indicate the path followed by the needle when inserted into the needle-guide (hyperechoic line).

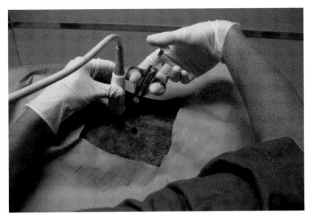

Figure 5.7 Performing a freehand biopsy.

from the injury. The biopsy is recommended when the subject can be monitored several hours after the procedure.

A number of factors affect the FNA and TCB diagnostic accuracy:

- For the FNA, the diagnostic quality of the sample is a factor, along with the underlying disease, since injuries have variable tendencies to release cellular material.
- For the TCB, the type of equipment used is a factor, along with the operator's experience and the injury type (necrosis/haemorrhage areas reduce chances of obtaining a definitive diagnosis).
- In any case, the diagnostic quality increases by collecting more samples.

TABLE 5.3 Where to take a sample (FNA or TCB)	
Location	
FOCAL INJURY	From the injury itself, avoiding haemorrhage/necrosis areas, if possible, as they would entail a non-diagnostic result. For this purpose, evaluating the injury vascularization by Doppler examination or echo-contrast agent is useful.
Diffuse injury	
LIVER	Sampling from left hepatic lobes is preferable, thus operating at greater distance from the gallbladder. With ascites and a small liver, doing a biopsy from peripheral portions of lobes which tend to move can be difficult, so a more cranial access through one intercostal space is preferable.
GALLBLADDER	The aspiration of gallbladder contents (cholecystocentesis) or from injuries of the gallbladder wall must be carried out, preferably crossing part of the liver parenchyma before entering the organ, so reducing any risk of bile leakage after the procedure.
KIDNEY	CORTEX: in case of diffuse renal disease, the cortex lateral portion of a renal pole must be used. The hilar region must be always avoided. The sampling must be performed from the renal cortex only, without penetrating the medullary. For a first rapid sample assessment, it can be placed on a slide, soaked with saline, then examined by microscopy. At 40X, acquired renal glomeruli (five complete glomeruli are needed, at least) can be counted. PELVIS If the renal pelvis is dilated, a urine sampling directly performed from the pelvis may be indicated; the sample is then physically evaluated, including the sediment analysis and/or the culture. In this case, a fine needle (preferably a 20–22 G spinal needle) is introduced and directed through the renal parenchyma until the pelvis is reached. This method is also useful to inject iodinated contrast agent, which allows for a contrastographic test (descending ureterography).
BLADDER	Injuries of the bladder wall can be easily aspirated transabdominally; however, this procedure must be avoided when a bladder carcinoma is suspected, due to the risk of metastatic seeding. An alternative method is aspiration by surgical catheterization (see below).

COMPLICATIONS

Complications related to bioptic procedures (FNA and TCB) vary depending on the following factors:

- Subject bleeding tendency (predisposition to coagulopathy, hypertension)
- Operator experience
- Examined organ (major complications for renal biopsies)
- Injury type
- Type of method used (lower with FNA versus the cutting-needle biopsy)
- Needle gauge.

Complications reported in the literature can be major and minor (Table 5.4).

SURGICAL CATHETERIZATION (ACCORDING TO LAMB 1996)

An ultrasound-assisted suction of the injury is performed. The catheter is introduced in the urinary tract until it reaches the injury (urethra or bladder); its position is checked on ultrasonography.

A strong suction is performed, aspirating several times with the catheter in maximum possible contact with the injury, also making slight back and forth motions, if necessary.

The catheter and the syringe are extracted as a whole, and cytology smears prepared using materials collected in the catheter (especially the tip). Sometimes, even small tissue frustules can be collected and sent for histopathological examination.

TABLE 5.4 Complications after FNA and TCB	
MINOR COMPLICATIONS: they are self-limiting and do not require any treatment. A variable 5–21% incidence was reported (Leveille 1993 and Bigge 2001).	Mild haemorrhage without decreased Hct. A small layer of perilesional effusion can be seen, which remains minimal and stable even a few minutes after the procedure. Within or close to the injury, a haematoma can be visualized as a homogeneous isoechoic/hypoechoic area that was not visible before the procedure.
	Tachycardia, polypnea, pale mucous membranes and increased capillary refill time (especially related to the pain if the procedure is done without sedation).
	For renal biopsies: microhematuria in 20–70% of cases * (self-limiting, it disappears within a few days, but must be monitored). Macroematuria: 1–4% of cases *. * Vaden 2005.
MAJOR COMPLICATIONS: They are rare and require urgent intervention (transfusions or surgery). A 1.2–6% incidence was reported (Leveille 1993 and Bigge 2001). For renal biopsies, higher values were reported (13.4 and 18.5% for dogs and cats, respectively, Vaden 2005).	Severe haemorrhage: the layer of perilesional effusion is abundant and increasing. Sometimes a hyperechoic jet can be seen going out of the bleeding vessel or body. In this case, the animal must be immediately monitored, checking repeatedly hematocrit and total protein.
	Gallbladder rupture and biliary peritonitis. This is especially associated to parietal necrosis areas, which should be identified before making the puncture. Around the gallbladder an effusion is visible that can be sampled to confirm the possible biliar origin. The risk of leakage of bile material from a normal gallbladder after aspiration is extremely low if the suction is performed transhepatically, since the liver parenchyma helps to close the small gap created.
	Septic peritonitis if abscesses are aspirated. In theory, a microbial dissemination within the abdominal cavity is possible, resulting in peritonitis. However, this event is very unlikely if the procedure was correctly performed, and can pose a real risk to the animal only in case of abscess rupture.
	Pancreatitis: it is possible, in theory, but actually the aspiration (FNA) of pancreatic tissue or cysts in this area is not associated to complications.
	Perirenal hematomas, hydronephrosis, retention cyst or arteriovenous fistulas (renal biopsies): the kidney appears to be the organ most prone to complications. This is another reason why thinner biopsy needles are preferred (18 G). The fluid therapy is crucial during and after the procedure to facilitate the removal of any clots.
	A pneumothorax is possible if lung biopsies are performed. In rare cases it occurs after ultrasonographic-assisted biopsies, if a solid injury in contact with the thoracic wall is sampled. If air amount is limited, the pneumothorax does not require any treatment.
	Metastatic seeding: reported for carcinomas, especially the transitional cell carcinoma of the urinary tract (Nylan 2002); metastases can lodge along the needle track. Therefore, the transabdominal aspiration must be avoided in case of suspected carcinoma of the urinary tract. Instead, the surgical catheterization technique must be used (Lamb 1996).

POSITIONING OF CATHETERS AND DRAINAGES (Fig. 5.8)

The introduction of catheters or drainages is facilitated by ultrasonographic assistance.

Drainages are positioned using a Seldinger technique and are designed to maintain the aspiration of cavities containing fluids or pus (cysts, abscesses).

Nephrostomic catheters may be useful to ensure a normal diuresis in subjects with hydronephrosis and obstruction of the lower urinary tract, pending definitive surgical treatments.

ALCOHOLIZATION OF CYSTS OR ABSCESSES

- It can be used to treat renal, liver and prostate cysts, or prostate abscesses
- 95% ethanol is used
- Volume to inject: about 30–40% of the aspirated fluid volume
- It is allowed to act for 10–15 minutes, possibly changing the subject position
- The alcohol must be aspirated and the cavity flushed with saline.

For alcoholization procedures note that:
- Sealing of the treated cavity must be checked, being sure there is no connection with the urethra or the renal pelvis
- The success rate of these procedures depends on the injury volume (often unsuccessful with large cysts or abscesses)
- They can be repeated 2/3 times at most; with further relapse, a different treatment is indicated
- They can cause complications: oedema and localized pain, tissue necrosis, fibrosis and neurinomas (reported in human medicine).

ULTRASONOGRAPHIC-ASSISTED INTRAOPERATIVE PROCEDURES

Using an intra-operative ultrasonographic system can be very useful to lead the surgeon to retrieve injuries or foreign bodies that are deeply located and hard to pinpoint solely by dissection. The ultrasonographic system must be properly prepared for use in the sterile field: the probe is covered with a sterile glove or probe cover, and cables are protected by sterile cable covers. Indications include:

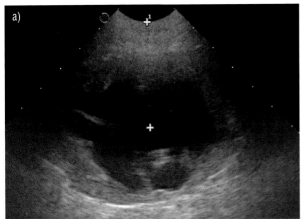

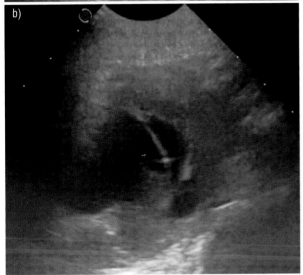

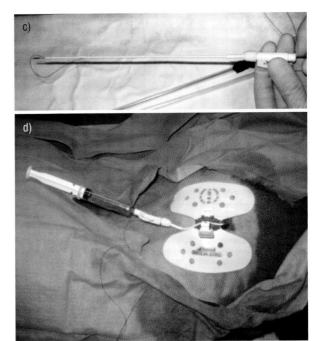

Figure 5.8   Positioning of a Dawson-Mueller 'pig tail' percutaneous drainage in the renal pelvis of a dog with complete urethral obstruction, bilateral hydronephrosis and severe renal failure **(a)**. Pending surgery that would repair the obstruction, a percutaneous drainage was introduced, allowing the subject to be kept under fluid therapy. **b)** The drainage entering the dilated pelvis is visualized. **c)** A detail of the used drainage. **d)** The drainage fixed on the dog's skin in the flank region will be subsequently connected to a closed urine collection system.

- Not directly visible brain or intramedullary neoplasms
- Intrahepatic portosystemic shunts located near the diaphragm
- Retrieval of deep foreign bodies (e.g. iliopsoas muscles). The surgical dissection is progressively led by visualizing the FB location. Sometimes, FBs can also be retrieved using an ultrasonographic-assisted direct access (non-surgical), using the fistula tract, or making a small skin dissection.

RECOMMENDED READING

Barr F: Percutaneous biopsy of abdominal organs under ultrasound guidance. JSAP 1995; 36: 105–113.

De Rycke LMJH, Van Bree H, Simoens PJM: Ultrasound-guided tissuecore biopsy of liver, spleen and kidney in normal dogs. Vet Rad & Ultrasound 1999; 40: 294–299.

Zatelli A, D'ippolito P, Zini E. Number and specimen length obtained from 100 dogs via percutaneous echo-assisted renal biopsy using two different needles. Vet Radio Ultrasound 2005; 46: 434–436.

Vaden SL, Levine JF, Lees GE, Groman RP, Grauer GF, Forrester SD. Renal biopsy: a retrospective study of methods and complications in 283 dogs and 65 cats. J Vet Intern Med 2005; 19: 794–801.

Leveille R, Partington BP, Biller DS, Miyabayashi T: Complications after ultrasound-guided biopsy of abdominal structures in dogs and cats: 246 cases (1984–1991), JAVMA 1993; 203: 413–415.

Bigge LA, Brown DJ, Pennick DG: Correlation between coagulation profile findings and bleedin complications after ultrasound-guided biopsies: 434 cases (1993–1996), JAAHA 2001; 37: 228–233.

Nylan TG, Wallack ST: Needle-tract implantation following us-guided FNA biopsy of transitional cell carcinoma of the bladder, urethra and prostate, Vet Rad & Ultr 2002.

Vignoli M, Rossi F, Chierici C, Terragni R, De Lorenzi D, Stanga M, Oliviero D: Neelde tract implantation after fine needle aspiration biopsy (FNAB) of transitional cell carcinoma of the urinary bladder and adenocarcinoma of the lung. Schweiz Arch Tierheilk 2007; 149: 314–318.

Lamb CR, Trower ND, Gregory SP: Ultrasound-guided catheter biopsy of the lower urinary tract: technique and results in 12 dogs. JSAP 1996; 37: 413–416.

Della Santa D, Rossi F, Carlucci F, Vignoli M, Kircher P Ultrasound-guided retrival of plant owns. Vet Radiol Ultr 2008; 49: 484–486.

6 Peritoneal cavity

Federica Rossi

SCAN TECHNIQUE

Animal preparation	• 12 hours on an empty stomach, at least. • Wide hair-clipping, including intercostal spaces. • Right and/or left lateral dorsal recumbency.
Probes	• Microconvex, 5 MHz mean frequency (3-7.5 MHz). • Linear, high-frequency (7.5-10 MHz) for small breed animals and to get details from small structures.
Scans and respective probe position	• To evaluate the peritoneum, the retroperitoneum and the serous membranes there are no reference fixed scans. • In case of suspected abdominal carcinomatosis, mainly in cats, it is recommended to scan all the abdomen with a high-frequency linear probe searching for peritoneal nodules adherent to the abdominal wall. • Peritoneal serous membranes are evaluated while examining various organs, observing the space that separates them and is interposed between the organs and the abdominal wall (Fig. 6.1). • On the contrary, the position of abdominal vessels is absolutely and/or relatively fixed to certain identifiable abdominal structures.

ULTRASONOGRAPHIC ANATOMY – GENERAL PERITONEAL CAVITY

Location	• All the abdomen.
Morphology, echostructure and echogenicity, edges	• The peritoneum appearance is strongly influenced by the amount of adipose tissue in the evaluated region. • The adipose tissue is mainly localized in the falciform ligament, the mesentery, the omentum, and the retroperitoneal space around the kidneys. It shows a typical coarse echostructure and is isoechoic/hyperechoic compared to the liver (Fig. 6.1). • If there is no adipose tissue, the peritoneal serous coat appears as a thin hyperechoic interface, with a smooth and regular surface (Fig. 6.1). • Normally, the abdomen contains 1.5 ml/kg of free fluid, but this is not visible on ultrasonography unless it reaches 2 ml kg. Puppies are an exception, and until six months a small amount of fluid is normally visible.

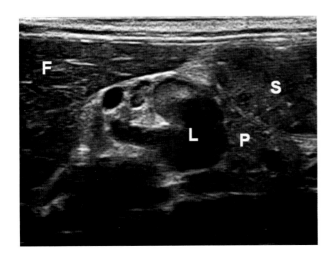

Figure 6.1 Optimal abdominal detail in a cat; examination with a linear probe. The adipose tissue that lies between the liver (F), the enlarged portal lymph node (L), the stomach (S), the pancreas (P) and vessels is well-defined and hyperechoic compared to adjacent structures. Organs are delimited by a smooth and regular, thin hyperechoic serous coat.

ABDOMINAL VESSELS

Location	The abdominal great vessels with their main tributary vessels must be identified.

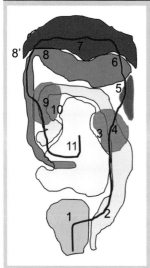	**AORTA (Ao) (Fig. 6.2, 6.3, 6.5 and 6.6):**
	• Cranially it lies dorsally, slightly to the left, then runs ventrally to the spine; before its end, it bifurcates into the two large external iliac arteries, then trifurcates into the two internal iliac arteries and the median sacral artery.
	• Following the Ao in the caudocranial direction (from position 2 in the cranial direction), the following tributary vessels can be identified:
	  – **External iliac aa. (Fig. 6.2 and 6.3c)**: they run in the caudolateral direction toward the ipsilateral limb, and have a lumen that is approximately 50% compared to the terminal Ao. They form an acute angle of about 30° as regards the Ao. It is almost never possible to obtain both external iliac arteries in the same image with the longitudinal scan, as they lie on different planes. Starting from the Ao, the two arteries can be separately followed directing the probe right and left. In the transverse scan instead, all vessels are simultaneously visible.
	  – **Deep iliac circumflex aa. (Fig. 6.3b)**: they have a small diameter and leave the Ao at right angles just cranially to the external iliac aa., at the site of medial iliac lymph nodes.
	  – **Caudal mesenteric aa.**: unpaired artery arising from the ventral surface of the Ao, just cranially to the previous ones; it is hard to visualize without the Colour Doppler.
	  – **Lumbar aa.**: paired arteries arising at regular distances between the iliac and renal aa.; they run dorsolaterally.
	  – **Ovarian or testicular aa.**: small sized, they are visible only in non neutered animals in the ovarian region, just caudally to the origin of renal aa.
	  – **Renal aa. (Fig. 6.3a)**: the left artery is more caudal. If examined with the animal in the right lateral recumbency and the scan performed from the left flank, at the origin it forms a well recognizable arc. The right artery branches more cranially. Note that about 20% of dogs have an accessory renal artery (Fig. 6.4). Renal arteries are coupled to their respective veins; the renal vein that goes with the artery is recognized for the larger diameter; moreover, it is more easily compressed, and moves towards the caudal vena cava.
	  – **Phrenicoabdominal aa.**: associated with the adrenal glands, they are small sized and run on the ventral surface of the gland. They are visible using the Doppler.
	  – **Cranial mesenteric and celiac aa. (Fig. 6.3a and 6.5)**: these two arteries arise from the Ao, just cranially to the left kidney, and run side by side in the first tract. This is why they are often visualized together as two tubular (longitudinal scan) or rounded (transverse scan) parallel structures. The cranial mesenteric artery runs mediocaudally, joining the mesenteric vein to then reach the root of mesentery. The **splenic, hepatic and left gastric aa.** arise from the celiac trunk; this trifurcation can be identified by following the celiac artery a few centimetres in the medial direction. Each of the three arteries can be followed to the periphery for a variable tract, according to the subject conditions (fed state, gastrointestinal content, sedated or awake animal).
	
	CAUDAL VENA CAVA (CVC) (Fig. 6.6 and 6.7):
	• It crosses the diaphragm slightly to the right of the mid-line, is located in the cranial abdomen ventrally to the Ao, and converges on the latter moving in the caudal direction. Its ending is adjacent to the Ao termination. The CVC identification requires a longitudinal scan of the middle/caudal abdomen, placing the probe just ventrally to the spine; here two vessels are visible (Ao and CVC) that tend to diverge in the cranial direction; the relative position of Ao and CVC depends on the selected recumbency: with the patient in the right lateral recumbency, the shallowest vessel is the Ao, while the deepest is the caudal vena cava. If the patient is in the left lateral recumbency, the shallowest vessel is the caudal vena cava, while the deepest is the Ao (Fig. 6.6). The CVC can be followed in the cranial direction up to the diaphragm (Fig. 6.7). Before the porta hepatis, the ascending and transverse colon containing fecal materials can make following the entire vessel path difficult. In this case, it is recommended going more cranially and finding the vessel again close to the liver.
	• It receives blood from suprahepatic veins.
	• Similar diameter to the Ao.

(Continued →)

ABDOMINAL VESSELS (Continued)

Location	• The CVC tributary veins correspond to arteries arising from the Ao described above; however, the anatomy of the venous system is less uniform. **PORTAL VEIN (PV) (Fig. 6.8, 6.9 and 6.10)** • It is localized ventrally and slightly to the right of the CVC. • It can be identified starting from the root of mesentery and following mesenteric veins in the cranial direction. These veins have progressively increasing diameters proceeding in the cranial direction, and converge to form the PV (Fig. 6.8 and 6.9). • Another option is using the right intercostal scan (position 8'), by placing the probe in one of the last intercostal spaces, just ventrally to the spine and just cranially to the cranial pole of the right kidney. Starting with a transverse scan, the ultrasound beam is directed slightly caudally to visualize part of the liver and the three vessels (aorta, vena cava and portal vein), the aorta dorsally, the vena cava slightly to the left, and the portal vein just caudally to the latter (Fig. 6.10). Having obtained this image, the probe is rotated to obtain a longitudinal scan of the portal vein at the porta hepatis. • Shortly before the porta hepatis, the PV performs a slight dorsal deviation (Fig. 6.9). • The diameter varies from 3.3 to 10.5 mm (dog) and from 3.4 to 5 mm (cat).
Morphology	• They appear as tubular structures in the longitudinal scan; roundish (arteries) or slightly oval (veins) structures in the transverse scan. • The veins shape varies depending on the compression exerted by the probe, while arteries keep a constant shape thanks to their thicker wall. • The PV has a more tortuous course compared to the CVC.
Relationships with adjacent organs evaluable on ultrasonography	They are surrounded by peritoneum and variable amounts of adipose tissue. Some vessels have direct relationships with groups of lymph nodes. In particular: • The external iliac arteries are adjacent to the medial iliac lymph nodes. • The mesenteric veins, at the root of mesentery, are in contact with jejunal lymph nodes. • Along the portal vein, the two hepatic lymph nodes are visualized at the porta hepatis. • In the adipose tissue that goes with the splenic vein the splenic lymph nodes are visualized.
Size	• The veins usually have a greater lumen compared to the corresponding arteries, and an easily compressible wall.
Edges	• Thin, smooth and regular.
Echogenicity	• Normally, the lumen is anechoic. In some subjects, especially if sedated and examined with high-resolution systems, a more echoic moving content inside the vessel is visible in some veins characterized by a particularly slow flow (more often, the splenic veins). • A thin and smooth hyperechoic wall, only visible where the ultrasound beam is perfectly perpendicular. • Be careful that the partial-volume artefact can create longitudinal echoes within the vessel. To differentiate them from a real structure, the vessel must be also evaluated in the transverse scan.
Echostructure	• Homogeneous.
Pulsed Wave (PW) Doppler	**Aorta and iliac circumflex aa., caudal mesenteric and lumbar aa. (Fig. 6.11a):** high-resistance pulsed flow characterized by: • A narrow and anterograde high-speed systolic peak (approaching flow). • Followed by a retrograde wave that corresponds to the first diastolic phase (moving away flow), at a lower speed compared to the first one. • A third approaching wave (second phase of the diastole), or a group of oscillatory waves with decreasing speed.

(Continued →)

ABDOMINAL VESSELS (Continued)

Pulsed Wave (PW) Doppler	**Renal aa., cranial mesenteric, celiac and their tributaries (Fig. 6.11b):** a medium-low resistance pulsed flow characterized by: • A broader high-speed systolic peak (approaching flow). • An approaching wave (diastolic) with lower speed compared to the previous one and progressively decreasing. • There is no retrograde wave. **CVC (see Fig. 7.3d, Chapter 7):** a flow characterized by a series of waves that reflect the right heart activity: • The first wider anterograde wave corresponds to the atrial systole. • The second small retrograde wave corresponds to the atrial filling. • The third anterograde wave corresponds to the opening of the atrioventricular valves and the passage of blood in the ventricle. • Other small waves are possible. • Additional speed variations are due to intrathoracic and intra-abdominal pressure changes that occur during breathing. During the inspiratory phase, the anterograde waves speed increases. **PV (see Fig. 7.3d, Chapter 7): Pulsed Wave (PW) Doppler:** an anterograde flow with a relatively uniform pattern and slight speed variations associated to the respiratory phase. The average speed of a normal flow is greater than 10 cm/s and lower than 20 cm/s. The main tributary veins of the portal vein are: • **Cranial and caudal mesenteric vv.:** visible in the middle abdomen near to the mesenteric artery, their convergence originates the portal vein. The caudal mesenteric vein is smaller and drains most of the caudal portion of the large intestine, while the cranial mesenteric drains most of the small intestine and the proximal segment of the large intestine. • **Splenic v.:** several parallel branches that drain all the spleen converge to the hilum and form the splenic vein that runs to the centre of the abdomen, where it goes caudally to the stomach and crosses the pancreas at the transition between the body and the left lobe. It receives the left gastric vein and enters the portal vein. • **Gastroduodenal v.:** a small vessel which runs along the gastric greater curvature. It drains the stomach, the duodenum and the pancreas. It is the last tributary of the portal vein before the porta hepatis.
Colour Doppler flow	• A homogeneously filled vessel lumen is visualized, whose colour is red (flow approaching the probe) or blue (flow moving away). With vessel turbulences, a colourful tessellated map is visible; the same happens if the Pulse Repetition Frequency (PRF) value is too low, or the Doppler gain is too high.

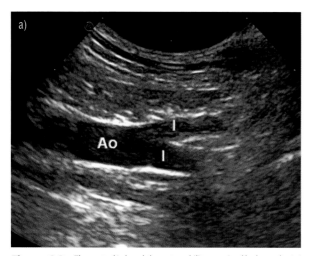 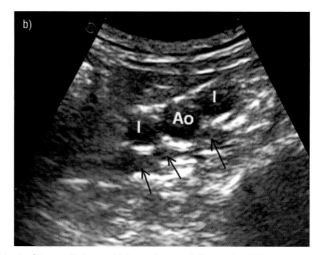

Figure 6.2 The aorta (Ao) and the external iliac arteries (I); the probe is in position 2. **a)** Longitudinal scan; this image shows both iliac arteries. **b)** Transverse scan; laterally to the Ao the two iliac arteries (I) are visible; more dorsally to the arteries, the corresponding iliac veins (arrows) are visible, partially collapsed.

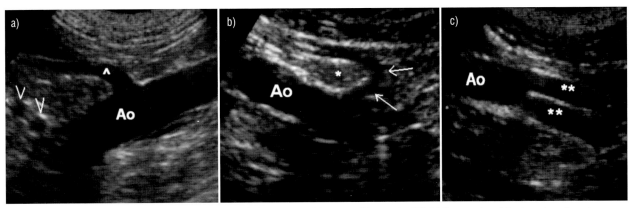

Figure 6.3 Ao examination in the caudocranial direction. **c)** The emersion of the external iliac arteries (**). **b)** The emersion of the deep circumflex artery (arrows), which borders the medial iliac lymph node (*). **a)** The emersion of the renal artery (^). A bit cranially, the cranial mesenteric and celiac aa. are visible in the transverse scan (V).

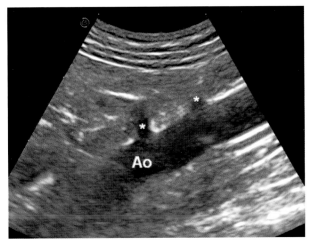

Figure 6.4 Longitudinal scan of the Ao performed from the left flank (position 3), caudomedially to the left kidney. In this dog two renal arteries (**) are showed; the main artery is more cranial, and the accessory artery is more caudal, both originating from the Ao.

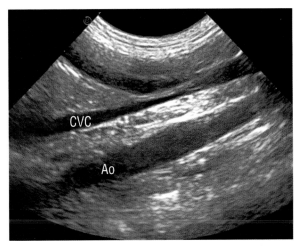

Figure 6.6 Longitudinal scan of Ao and CVC performed from the right flank. The CVC is more ventral, and the lumen slightly compressed due to the probe pressure. The Ao, more dorsal, maintains a more constant lumen. Cranially, the two vessels tend to diverge.

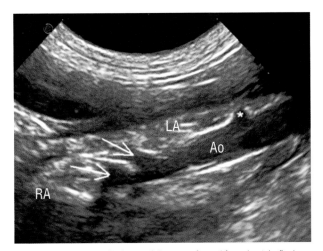

Figure 6.5 Longitudinal scan of the Ao performed from the right flank; some arteries arising from the Ao are visible. More cranially, the two paired cranial mesenteric and celiac arteries (arrows) are identifiable, while caudally the renal artery (*) is visible. These landmarks are important to localize the adrenal glands and possibly their injuries; the right adrenal gland (RA) is located cranially to the paired arteries, while the left gland (LA) lies between them and the renal artery.

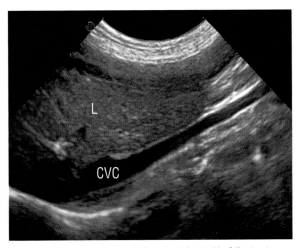

Figure 6.7 Longitudinal scan of the CVC obtained by following its course by a ventral approach, slightly to the right (position 10). In this dog, the CVC can be followed for a long tract in the cranial direction until its intra-hepatic portion. L = liver.

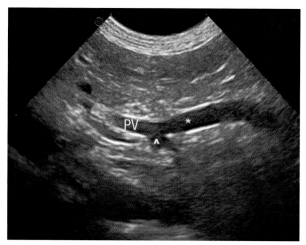

Figure 6.8 Middle-central abdomen; the image shows the origin of the PV, which rises from the confluence of the cranial mesenteric (*) and the caudal mesenteric (^) veins.

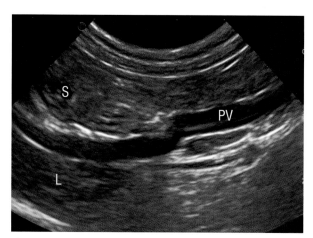

Figure 6.9 Longitudinal scan of the portal vein obtained by a ventral approach, slightly oriented to the right. The portal vein, just caudally to the porta hepatis, deviates dorsally. L = liver. S = stomach.

PERITONEAL DISEASES OF ULTRASONOGRAPHIC INTEREST

The most common peritoneal diseases of ultrasonographic interest are:

- Abdominal effusion
- Pneumoperitoneum
- Peritonitis
- Neoplasm

ABDOMINAL EFFUSION (Table 6.1)

The ultrasonography is more sensitive compared to radiology in detecting abdominal fluid and enables the visualization of the smallest effusions (Fig. 6.12).

The literature (Henley 1989) reports 2 ml/kg of fluid as the smallest amount of effusion to be visible; currently, this limit is surpassed by the availability of high-resolution systems.

- The effusion facilitates the exploration of the peritoneal serous coat (Fig. 6.13 and 6.14) that must be carefully studied

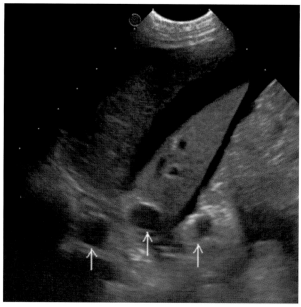

Figure 6.10 Right intercostal scan (position 8') with the probe oriented in the caudal direction. The three arrows indicate, from left to right, the Ao, the CVC and the PV. In this dog, the anechoic effusion eases the visualization of hepatic lobes and vessels.

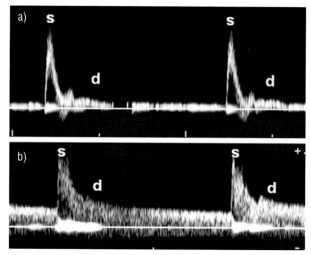

Figure 6.11 Pulsed Wave (PW) Doppler of a high-resistance **(a)** and a low-resistance **(b)** artery. **a)** Ao: the high-resistance flow features a narrow systolic peak, a short retrograde wave and a third approaching wave. **b)** Low-resistance flow (renal a.), with a wider high-speed systolic peak and a speed of the diastolic wave that is lower compared to the previous one and progressively decreasing; s = systole, d = diastole.

for possible nodules (which may direct towards a diagnosis of neoplasm) or other injuries (abscesses, foreign bodies).

- It should be emphasized that the mere presence of an effusion increases the echogenicity and visibility of the peritoneal adipose tissue, due to the posterior-wall enhancement created by the fluid (Fig. 6.15). Therefore, especially in animals with abundant peritoneal fat, it can be difficult to differentiate the normal adipose tissue from the real thickening and/or hyperechogenicity of the peritoneum, associated for example to the peritonitis (Fig. 6.17). To find one's way, it is important to understand:
  - If the hyperechoic appearance is uniform throughout the abdominal cavity or more evident in some areas,

which could be the source of the problem (for example, a perforation of the gastrointestinal tract or a peritoneal abscess)
- If there is a distal echoes dispersion. The different molecular composition of inflamed tissues creates a hyperechogenicity associated with 'image blurring'. Edges are not well-defined, the abdominal detail disappears, and images are very deteriorated. On the contrary, in adipose tissues that are hyperechoic due to posterior-wall enhancement, the same image deterioration is not shown, edges remain clear-cut, and the detail intact.
- It is essential searching for other signs of abdominal inflammation (adjacent-bowel wrinkling, pancreatic changes, associated focal peritoneal injuries).

PNEUMOPERITONEUM (Table 6.1)

After laparotomy or abdominal trauma, free gas can be visible and persist for several days. After a surgery, the gas amount decreases exponentially during the first 14 days, but gas traces can be detected even after four weeks.

Other causes of pneumoperitoneum include rupture of a hollow organ (primarily the gastrointestinal tract, but the bladder was also reported), necrosis of a parenchyma (spleen) or a peritonitis with gas-producing bacteria (Clostridia, rare occurrence).

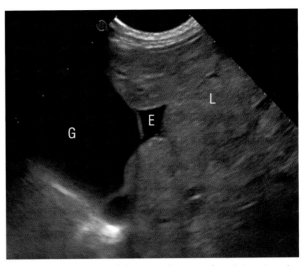

Figure 6.12 This animal shows a small amount of anechoic peritoneal effusion (E), which accumulates between the gallbladder (G) and the liver parenchyma (L). The liver is heterogeneous, with irregular edges, and the dog had a severe liver cirrhosis.

Free gas in the abdominal cavity can be difficult to visualize from an ultrasonographic point of view, especially for inexperienced operators. In doubtful cases, the radiographic examination can help (the horizontal-beam view is more accurate).

TABLE 6.1 - Ultrasonographic features of various types of abdominal collections		
Amount and type of collection	**Location**	**Ultrasonographic appearance**
Small collection of free fluid (Fig. 6.12 and 6.14)	Especially visible in dependent portions of the abdomen (accumulated by gravity); with the animal in the lateral recumbency, after a few minutes the fluid is more easily visualized by placing the probe in the most ventral portions, especially near the bladder or between the hepatic lobes. Other locations to check are those adjacent to the spleen (left lateral edge) and between the intestinal loops. An excessive pressure on the probe must be avoided, which would move the effusion elsewhere.	The echogenicity of a fluid collection varies from a uniform anechoic appearance to a fluid rich in hyperechoic foci, depending on the cellular content. The greater the cellularity, the higher the echogenicity: • The less cellular effusions (e.g. transudate due to heart disease or hypoalbuminemia, urine, chyle) are anechoic or hypoechoic (Fig. 6.12–15) • Modified transudates, exudates and haemorrhagic effusions have a mobile corpuscular component that can make them greatly echoic, like a parenchyma (Fig. 6.16). • Especially with a chronic purulent infection, possible findings are septa or fibrin build-ups that tend to make the effusion more echoic and heterogeneous (Fig. 6.17). • If the effusion is haemorrhagic, peritoneal hematomas may form whose echogenicity may vary over time depending on the stage of clot reorganization. The haematoma appears initially as a homogeneous hyperechoic mass; then, it acquires a more heterogeneous appearance with anechoic cavities and septa.
Abundant collection of free fluid (Fig. 6.13 and 6.15)	Visible everywhere, it separates the abdominal organs.	
Saccate fluid collection	In this case, it does not respond to the law of gravity and maintains its position regardless of the animal recumbency.	
Small collection, gaseous only	If free, it tends to become localized, by gravity, in the most dorsal abdominal regions, accumulating between the non-declivous abdominal wall and the underlying abdominal organs.	It is necessary to search for an echogenic interface characterized by the production of typical gas artefacts (reverberations, comet tail); this interface is localized just below the abdominal wall, and is not contained within a portion of the gastrointestinal tract. To avoid any confusion with the gas contained in the intestinal lumen, it is recommended to look for the gas collection near a parenchyma (for example, with the dog in the right lateral recumbency, the region between the left abdominal wall and the surface of the spleen or a liver lobe).
Abundant gas collection	The gas is distributed between the organs, making their visualization difficult due to artefacts (reverberation, shadowing) created by the gas.	
Gas collection, associated to fluid	Variable.	The gas can mix, forming small hyperechoic foci and creating the ring-down artefact.

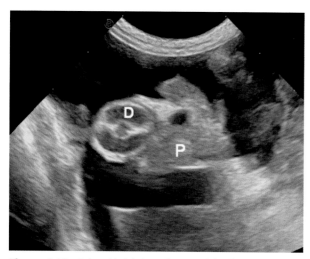

Figure 6.13 A dog with right heart disease and abundant anechoic effusion. The effusion surrounds and reveals the edges of the peritoneal serous coat (usually invisible), which marks off the duodenum (D) and the pancreas (P), and appears thin, smooth and regular.

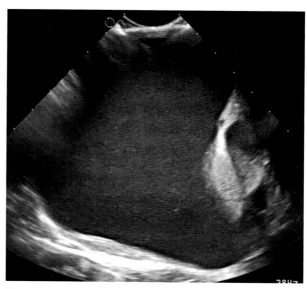

Figure 6.16 Haemorrhagic retroperitoneal effusion, which appears strongly echoic due to an abundant corpuscular component.

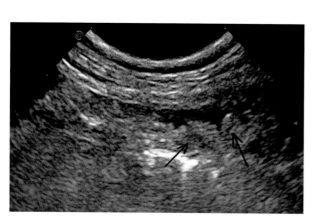

Figure 6.14 A small amount of anechoic effusion, which reveals the thickened peritoneum, with irregular surface and small metastatic nodules (carcinomatosis).

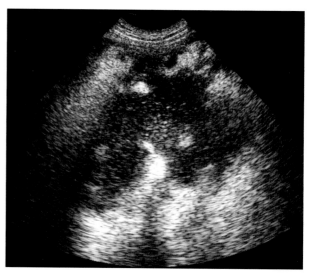

Figure 6.17 A dog with septic effusion and peritonitis. The effusion is corpuscular, and the peritoneum appears hyperechoic. The echooes distal dispersion creates image blurring, with poor definition of the underlying serous membranes.

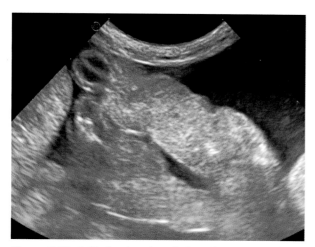

Figure 6.15 In this dog, the peritoneal adipose tissue appears markedly hyperechoic; this appearance is due to an abundant anechoic effusion (posterior-wall enhancement). The edges of the visible structures are clearly defined, and the detail is optimal.

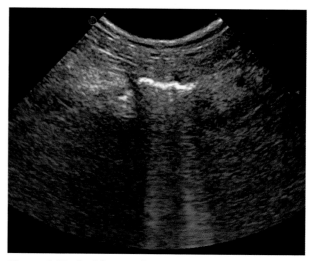

Figure 6.18 Small free gas collection in peritoneum with the typical appearance of hyperechoic interface associated with reverberation. The adjacent peritoneum is hyperechoic, ill-defined.

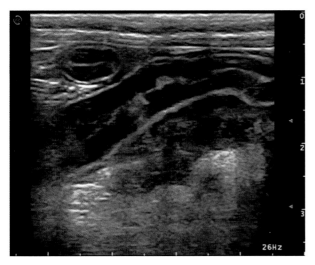

Figure 6.19 Pancreatitis and peritonitis in a dog. The pancreas is enlarged and hypoechoic, while the adjacent mesentery is hyperechoic; this causes distal echoes dispersion that blurs the image in the far field. The duodenal wall is thickened and the lumen slightly dilated.

PERITONITIS AND STEATITIS (Fig. 6.17 and 6.19)

Inflammation of the peritoneal cavity can affect the peritoneal serous coat (peritonitis) and/or the mesenteric adipose tissue (steatitis). Among the causes, we must remember infections of the abdominal cavity (FIP, sepsis from intestinal perforation, or FB migration), and non-infectious inflammatory diseases (e.g. secondary to pancreatitis or biliary tract rupture). In dogs a form of idiopathic steatitis (Komori 2002) was also reported, that involved the mesenteric adipose tissue and the gastros-plenic ligament.

Ultrasonographic findings of peritonitis and steatitis include:

- Effusion, more or less rich in echoic foci. Echogenicity varies depending on cellular content, then on the cause; the appearance is hypoechoic e.g. in the FIP, while it is hyperechoic in the case of purulent or haemorrhagic effusion (see Table 6.1)
- Thickening and hyperechogenicity of the mesentery
- Greater attenuation and distal echoes dispersion (scattering) by the mesenteric fat, which reduces the visualization of underlying organs
- Free air possible, especially with intestinal perforation
- The lesion may be widespread (e.g. FIP) or more focused if there is a specific cause (e.g. pancreatitis, intestinal focal injury).

NODULAR NECROSIS OF PERITONEAL ADIPOSE TISSUE

Accidental finding, most common in cats, especially obese subjects. There are areas of nodular necrosis of the adipose tissue, not associated with changes in the surrounding peritoneum.

Well-defined hyperechoic nodules are visible, located in the mesenteric adipose tissue or the omentum. If mineralized, they are associated with clean posterior acoustic shadow.

ABSCESSES/GRANULOMAS/FOREIGN BODIES (FBs)

Abscesses or granulomas can be caused by bacterial, fungal, or viral (FIP) infections, or by FBs (e.g. vegetable foreign bodies, bones or wood fragments migrated from the gastrointestinal system, or surgical gauzes).

Abscesses (Fig. 6.20) appear as oval/rounded injuries; the most typical appearance is an injury bounded by a hyperechoic capsule filled with fluid and possibly with gas. As an alternative, they appear diffusely hypoechoic or complex-type.

Granulomas (Fig. 6.21) have a more solid appearance, even though they may be associated with cavities filled with fluid, or fistulas.

Fistulas appear as hypoechoic tracts that feature a lumen filled with fluid or gas, and go for example from the skin to the depths. In dogs, fistulas are quite common in the flank region; they are due to vegetable FBs that migrate, often in the retroperitoneal region. In these cases, ultrasonography may be useful to identify the FB and facilitate its removal by means of ultrasonography-assisted surgery. To identify the FB, the sublumbar

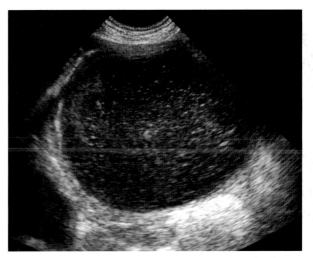

Figure 6.20 Peritoneal abscess presenting a thick wall and abundant corpuscular hyperechoic content.

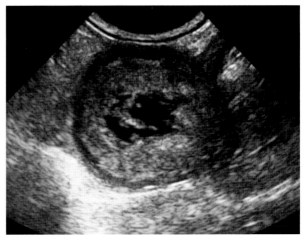

Figure 6.21 Peritoneal granuloma (secondary to intestinal perforation) with thick hyperechoic capsule and poor hypoechoic content.

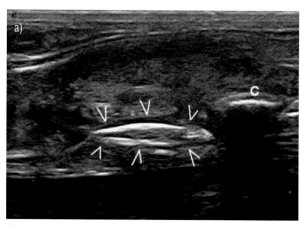
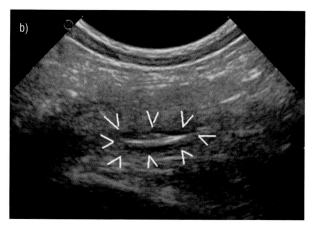

Figure 6.22 Examples of vegetable FBs found on ultrasonography (delimited by arrowheads). **a)** The FB was located inside the thoracic wall, adjacent to a rib (C) and surrounded by thickened tissue. **b)** Small vegetable FB visualized inside the iliopsoas muscle.

region is explored following the fistula tracts, and searching for a linear structure that includes a double hyperechoic interface that almost never produces shadowing.

Under ideal conditions, the FB is easily identified and recognized, but in the real world these cases are a challenge even for the most experienced ultrasonographers. The factors that complicate the evaluation include:

1. The time elapsed from the entrance of the FB and the ultrasonographic examination: if performed months or even years after the disease onset, the FB is difficult to identify because it is probably macerated, losing morphological characteristics that help its identification.
2. The type of surrounding tissue: if the FB is localized within an abscess or surrounded by an anechoic effusion, it is more easily recognizable because it differs from surrounding tissues; in contrast, if it is contained within a muscle belly or a hyperechoic granuloma, it is very difficult to visualize.
3. The localization of the foreign body: the typical localization is the sublumbar region, ventrally to the lumbar vertebral bodies (L2 and L3); the FB migrates here

after it is aspired, and crosses the respiratory tract, the lungs and the diaphragm. Respiratory acts move the EC in the caudal direction along the pillars of the diaphragm until its insertion in the sublumbar position. The FB can theoretically sit at any point on the way, although it is often found within the iliopsoas muscle. The more cranial the location, the greater the difficulty to find it on ultrasonography, due to increased thickness of interposed soft tissues.

Another type of peritoneal FB that can be found in small animals is a surgical gauze (left behind during previous surgery), which appears as a hypoechoic mass with an irregular hyperechoic centre.

PERITONEAL NEOPLASM

It may be primary or metastatic (carcinomatosis). Primary neoplasms include simple or infiltrating lipomas, liposarcomas, hemangiosarcomas or other sarcomas, and the mesothelioma.

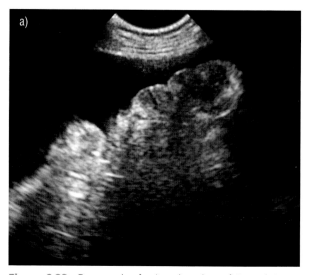
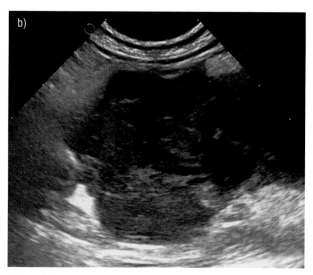

Figure 6.23 Two examples of peritoneal neoplasm. **a)** Hyperechoic mass associated with effusion (liposarcoma). **b)** Hypoechoic mass surrounded by hyperechoic peritoneum (fibrosarcoma).

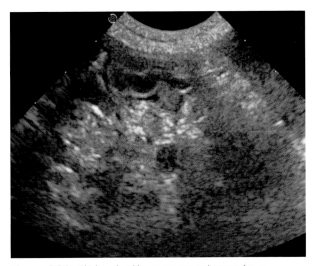

Figure 6.24 Thickened and heterogeneous peritoneum due to hypoechoic nodular injuries (metastases from splenic haemangiosarcoma).

They appear as hyperechoic or heterogeneous masses. Lipomas have the typical appearance of adipose tissue, are hyperechoic and associated with echoes attenuation. Hemangiosarcomas, quite common in the retroperitoneum, can show a complex mass pattern, and overrun adjacent great vessels (vena cava, renal veins, aorta).

Peritoneal carcinomatosis is caused by metastatic dissemination of primary abdominal neoplasms, most often carcinomas of the gastrointestinal tract (cat) or the haemangiosarcoma (dog).

Ultrasonographic findings include:

- Peritoneal effusion
- Irregular thickening of peritoneum
- Presence of nodules, often hypoechoic compared to the mesenteric adipose tissue. Previous findings are compatible with peritonitis, but finding nodules is very important to move towards an oncological disease; therefore, if carcinomatosis is suspected, it is important to carefully examine the peritoneal surface adjacent to effusion layers, where nodules are easier to identify
- Lymphadenopathy.

RECOMMENDED READING

Hanley RK, Hager DA, Ackerman N. A comparison of two-dimensional ultrasonography and radiography for the detection of small amounts of free peritoneal fluid in the dog. Vet Rad & Ultrasound, 1989; 30:121–124.

Spaulding KA. Sonographic evaluation of peritoneal effusion in small animals. Vet Rad & Ultraspund 1993; 34:427–431.

Komori S, Nakagaki K, Koyama H, Yamagami T. Idiopathic mesenteric and omental steatitis in a dog. J Am Vet Med Assoc. 2002; 221:1591–1593.

Boysen SR, Tidwell AS, Penninck D. Ultrasonographic findings in dogs and cats with gastrointestinal perforation. Vet Rad & Ultrasound 2003; 44:556–564.

Della Santa D, Rossi F, Carlucci F, Vignoli M, Kircher P Ultrasound-guided retrieval of plant awns. Vet Rad & Ultrasound Ultras 2008; 49(5): 484–486.

Merlo M, Lamb CR. Radiographic and ultrasonographic features of retained surgical sponge in eight dogs. Vet Rad & Ultrasound Ultras 2000; 41(3):279–283.

Penninck D, Mitchell SL. Ultrasonographic detection of ingested and perforating wooden foreign bodies in four dogs. J Am Vet Med Assoc. 2003; 223(2):206–209.

Schwarz T, Morandi F, Gnudi G, Wisner E, Paterson C, Sullivan M, Johnston P. Nodular fat necrosis in the feline and canine abdomen. Vet Rad & Ultrasound 2000; 41(4):335–339.

Monteiro CB, O'Brien RT A retrospective study on the sonographic findings of abdominal carcinomatosis in 14 cats. Vet Rad & Ultrasound 2004; 45(6):559–564.

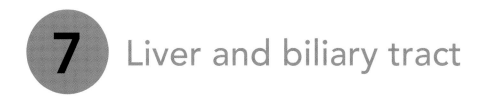

7 Liver and biliary tract

Federica Rossi

SCAN TECHNIQUE (Fig. 7.1)

Animal preparation	• 12 hours on an empty stomach, at least. • Wide hair-clipping, including intercostal spaces. • Right and/or left lateral dorsal recumbency.
Probes	• Microconvex, 5 MHz mean frequency (3–7.5 MHz). • Linear, high-frequency (7.5–10 MHz), for small breed animals and organ surface portions.
Scans and respective probe position 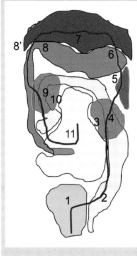	• **Longitudinal scan** (position 7, Fig. 7.1a): the probe is in contact with the xyphoid process of the sternum, the beam is oriented longitudinally and in the craniodorsal direction, to explore the part of the liver delimited by the costal arch. Starting from a median position, move right and left following the costal arch. To the left, the visualization can be obstructed by the stomach (especially if distended with gas); in this case switch to the intercostal scan. • **Transverse scan** (position 7, Fig. 7.1b): the probe is in contact with the xyphoid process of the sternum, rotated by 90° compared to the longitudinal scan; the beam is oriented transversally and in the craniodorsal direction with variable obliquity, so the organ can be explored from the diaphragm to the porta hepatis. • **Oblique scans** (Fig. 7.1c, d): the probe moves from position 7 to position 6 and 8, sliding along the costal arch and being tilted to left and right. • **Intercostal scans** (positions 6' and 8', Fig. 7.1e, f): the probe is over the last two intercostal spaces, allowing for the visualization of lateral lobes localized caudally to the lungs and the quadrate lobe (on the right). Among these scans, the oblique scan obtained from the right is very important (Fig. 7.1f) as the three abdominal vessels (aorta, caudal vena cava and portal vein) can be visualized. To obtain this scan, the probe is placed over one of the last intercostal spaces, slightly ventral to the spine and just cranially to the cranial pole of the right kidney; starting with a transverse scan, the ultrasound beam is directed slightly caudally, to show part of the liver and the three vessels in the transverse scan (Fig. 7.2d). Having obtained this image, vessels can be followed in the cranial and caudal direction, slightly tilting the probe.

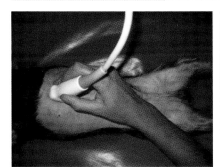

Figure 7.1a   Position 7, liver longitudinal scan.

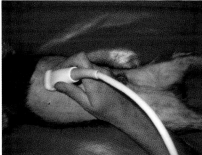

Figure 7.1b   Position 7, liver transverse scan.

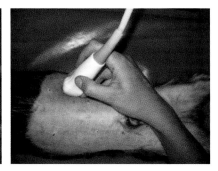

Figure 7.1c   Position 6, oblique scan directed on the left.

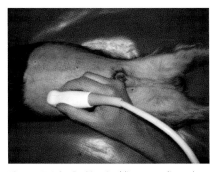

Figure 7.1d   Position 8, oblique scan directed on the right.

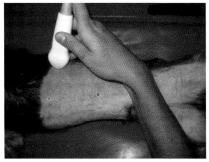

Figure 7.1e   Position 6, left intercostal scan.

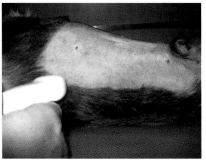

Figure 7.1f   Position 8, right intercostal scan.

ULTRASONOGRAPHIC ANATOMY – LIVER (Fig. 7.2 and 7.3)

Location	• Middle, right and left, cranial abdomen.
Morphology	• **Six lobes:** left and right, left medial and right medial, quadrate, caudate (divided into caudate and papillary processes). • Normally, interlobar fissures are not visible. • The gallbladder separates the quadrate lobe from the right medial lobe. • It is disrupted by vascular structures.
Relationships with adjacent organs evaluable on ultrasonography	• **Cranially:** hyperechoic acoustic interface separating the diaphragm and the lung (ATTENTION to the mirror effect). • **Caudally to the left:** gastric fundus, peritoneal adipose tissue, spleen (only with not distended stomach). • **Caudally to the right:** pylorus and duodenum, right lobe of the pancreas, caudate lobe in contact with the cranial pole of the right kidney. • **Ventrally**: adipose tissue of the falciform ligament (BE CAREFUL to not confuse it with the liver parenchyma in obese subjects).
Size	• **Subjective evaluation:** • Consider the distance between the diaphragm and the stomach (left) and between the diaphragm and the right kidney (right); • Assess the size relationship between the liver and the gallbladder (in case of microhepatia, the gallbladder appears larger); • In case of hepatomegaly, edges are rounded (Fig. 7.2f) and the caudal portion of hepatic lobes reaches and sometimes exceeds the gastric fundus (left) and the right kidney (right).
Si Edges (Fig. 2e, f)	• Thin, smooth and regular. • Sharp apex of the hepatic lobes
Mean	• Echogenicity • Hypoechoic compared to the spleen (Fig. 7.2g). • Isoechoic or slightly hyperechoic compared to the renal cortex (Fig. 7.2h). • Isoechoic or slightly hypoechoic compared to the adipose tissue of the falciform ligament.

(Continued →)

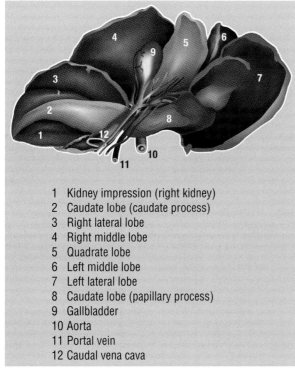

1 Kidney impression (right kidney)
2 Caudate lobe (caudate process)
3 Right lateral lobe
4 Right middle lobe
5 Quadrate lobe
6 Left middle lobe
7 Left lateral lobe
8 Caudate lobe (papillary process)
9 Gallbladder
10 Aorta
11 Portal vein
12 Caudal vena cava

Figure 7.2a Schematic of the gross anatomy of the liver with six lobes.

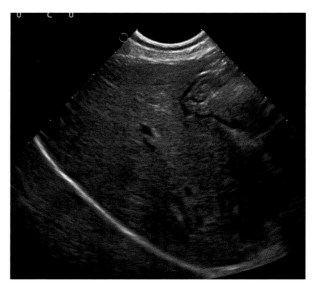

Figure 7.2b Dog, normal liver, longitudinal scan.

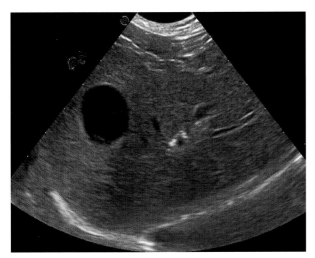

Figure 7.2c   Dog, normal liver, transverse scan.

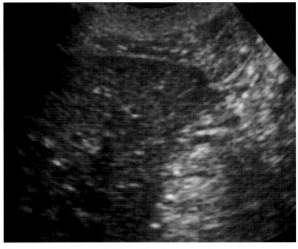

Figure 7.2f   Dog, rounded liver edges, hepatomegaly.

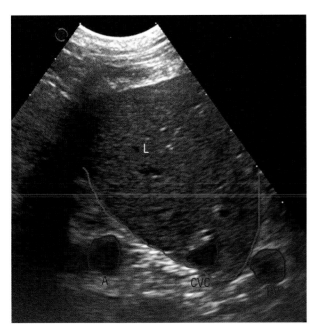

Figure 7.2d   Dog, normal liver, oblique right intercostal scan. A = aorta CVC = caudal vena cava, PV = portal vein, L = liver.

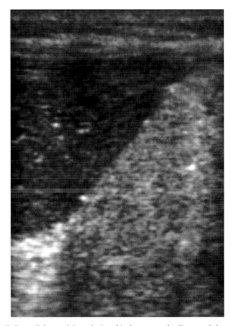

Figure 7.2g   Echogenicity relationship between the liver and the spleen (the liver parenchyma is less echoic compared to the spleen).

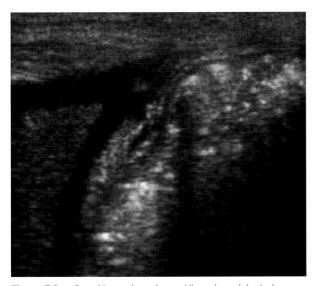

Figure 7.2e   Dog, thin, regular and normal liver edges, abdominal effusion.

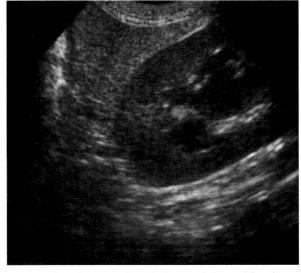

Figure 7.2h   Echogenicity relationship between the liver and the right kidney (the liver parenchyma is more echoic compared to the renal cortex).

ULTRASONOGRAPHIC ANATOMY – LIVER (Continued)

Echostructure	• Homogeneous. • Slightly coarser than the spleen. • Finer compared to adipose tissue of the adjacent falciform ligament.
Vessels	**Caudal vena cava (CVC)** (Fig. 7.3a, Fig. 6.6 and 6.7, Chapter 6) • Anechoic tubular structure with straight course; running through the dorsal portion of the liver, it crosses the diaphragm slightly to the right of the mid-line. To identify the CVC, start with a longitudinal scan of the medio-central abdomen; here you see two vessels (aorta and CVC) that tend to diverge in the cranial direction; the most ventral vessel is the CVC, which may be followed cranially until the dorsal edge of the liver and the diaphragm. Before the porta hepatis, the ascending and transverse colon containing the fecal material can make it difficult to follow the entire vessel path. In this case, it is recommended going more cranially and finding the vessel again close to the liver. • It receives blood from suprahepatic veins. • Similar diameter to the aorta. • Easily compressible lumen. • Pulsed Wave (PW) Doppler: a flow that moves away (below the baseline) with three waves reflecting activities of the right heart (Fig. 7.3d). **Portal vein (PV)** (Fig. 7.3b) • Ventrally and slightly to the right of the CVC. It can be identified starting from the root of mesentery and following mesenteric veins in the cranial direction. These veins merge to create the PV, whose diameter progressively increases proceeding in a cranial direction. Shortly before the porta hepatis, the PV makes a slight dorsal deviation (Fig. 6.9, Chapter 6). • More tortuous course compared to the CVC. • The diameter varies from 3.3 to 10.5 mm (dog) and from 3.4 to 5 mm (cat). • It divides into right (smaller) and left (larger) branches. • Pulsed Wave (PW) Doppler: a linear flow that moves away (below the baseline); speed changes are associated to respiration phases (Fig. 7.3d). **Intrahepatic veins** (Fig. 7.3c) • **Suprahepatic veins:** anechoic tubular structures that converge toward the CVC; very thin and normally invisible wall. • **Portals branches:** anechoic tubular structures that diverge from the portal vein, separated by hyperechoic interface ('wall')*. Hepatic arteries: • Extrahepatic portions of hepatic aa. are only identifiable using the Doppler function at the porta hepatis. • Pulsed Wave (PW) Doppler flow represents the typical pulsed arterial flow that is approaching the probe (above the baseline).
Tributary lymph nodes	• **Hepatic or portals.** • **Gastric.** • **Splenic.**

*The so-called 'wall' described for intrahepatic portal branches is not a real vascular wall, but an interface made by the connective tissue that surrounds structures that form the so-called portal triad (one portal vein branch, one hepatic artery branch and the bile duct), located between the liver lobules.

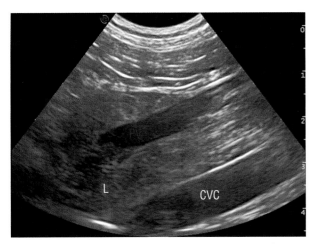

Figure 7.3a CVC and PV in the longitudinal scan, near the porta hepatis. The CVC is more dorsal and moves towards the diaphragm hyperechoic interface, coming into contact with the liver (L) dorsal portion.

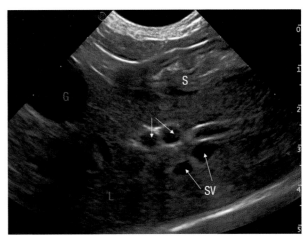

Figure 7.3c Transverse scan of the liver where the PV separates in its two main branches, right and left (PV). More dorsally, the two suprahepatic veins (SV) are visible; unlike the PV, their wall is not delimited by a hyperechoic interface. L = liver, S = stomach, G = gallbladder.

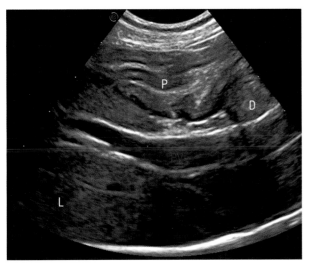

Figure 7.3b PV, longitudinal scan where it separates into intrahepatic portal branches. The origin of the right portal branch is visible, where the PV diameter is reduced. P = pyloric antrum, D = duodenum, L = liver.

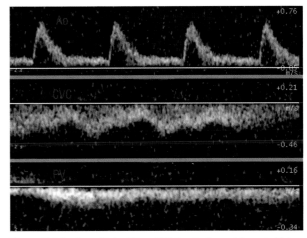

Figure 7.3d Normal Pulsed Wave (PW) Doppler flows of the aorta (Ao), the caudal vena cava (CVC) and the portal vein (PV). Ao: typical flow of an artery with systolic peak and low-speed diastolic flow. CVC: three-phase flow moving away from the baseline and reflecting the cardiac activity of the right heart. PV: low-speed flow that is moving away, with slight changes caused by the respiratory activity.

ULTRASONOGRAPHIC ANATOMY – GALLBLADDER (G) AND EXTRAHEPATIC BILIARY TRACT (BT) (Fig. 7.4)

Location	G: right cranial abdomen.
	BT: from the gallbladder in the caudal direction they reach the duodenum to flow into the major duodenal papilla (dog and cat) and/or the minor duodenal papilla (dog).
Morphology	G: piriformis (longitudinal scan) or rounded (transverse scan) (Fig. 7.4a and b). In cats, anatomical variants (bipartite gallbladder or double gallbladder with septa) are not uncommon (Fig. 7.4c).
	BT: the cystic duct, continuation of the 'C' neck, receives hepatic ducts and becomes the common bile duct (CBD). The CBD ends in the major duodenal papilla and is visible, especially in cats, at the porta hepatis as tubular structure with a sometimes tortuous course, that runs craniocaudally from the liver to the duodenum.
	The major duodenal papilla is also the termination of the pancreatic duct. There is a difference between dogs and cats: sphincters of the two ducts are separated in dogs, while they converge in their distal portion in cats (Fig. 7.4d). Note that the dog has an accessory pancreatic duct (which, despite its name, is the larger diameter duct) that opens in the minor duodenal papilla. The anatomy of this region is not always constant even in individuals of the same species.

(Continued →)

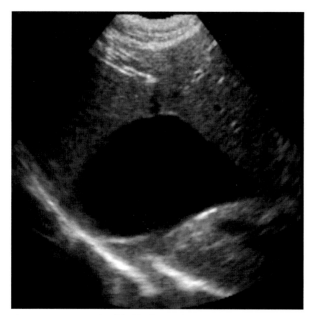

Figure 7.4a Normal gallbladder, longitudinal scan.

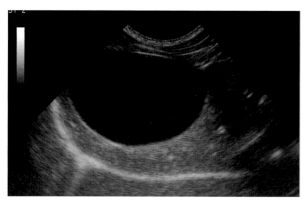

Figure 7.4b Normal gallbladder, transverse scan.

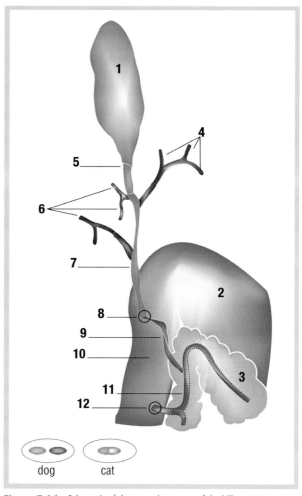

Figure 7.4d Schematic of the normal anatomy of the biliary tract.
1 = gallbladder – 2 = pyloric part of the stomach – 3 = pancreas – 4 and 6 = hepatic ducts – 5 = cystic duct – 7 = bile duct – 8 = major duodenal papilla – 9 = pancreatic duct – 10 = duodenum – 11 = accessory pancreatic duct – 12 = minor duodenal papilla

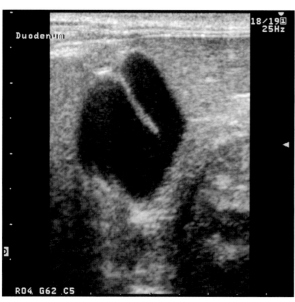

Figure 7.4c Bipartite gallbladder in a cat.

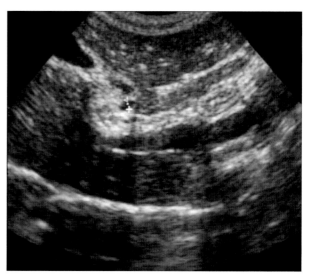

Figure 7.4e Cursors mark off the normal CBD in a cat, located just ventrally to the portal vein.

ULTRASONOGRAPHIC ANATOMY – GALLBLADDER (C) AND EXTRAHEPATIC BILIARY TRACT (BT) (Continued)

Relationships with adjacent organs evaluable on ultrasonography	**G:** quadrate lobe (left) and right medial lobe (right), peritoneal adipose tissue caudally, sometimes in contact with the diaphragm cranially. **BT:** liver parenchyma, peritoneum, pancreas, duodenum (in a craniocaudal direction).
Size	**G:** variable according to fasting period; in anorexic animals can be very distended. Such ultrasonographic finding is therefore not indicative of biliary obstruction. BT: maximum CBD diameter: 3 mm (dog), 4 mm (cat). In cats, CBD is more visible compared to dogs (bigger normal diameter). **NB:** normally, intrahepatic ducts are not visible.
Wall	**G:** thin, hyperechoic, with uniform thickness of 2–3 mm (dog) and 1 mm (cat) BT: hyperechoic, thin and smooth.
Echogenicity	**G:** anechoic content; normally, modest amounts of sediment (sludge) in dogs; the anechoic content produces intense posterior-wall enhancement. Attention to the lateral acoustic shadows artefact, associated with convex lateral edges of the organ. **BT:** anechoic lumen.

ULTRASONOGRAPHY IN LIVER DISEASES

The ultrasonographic examination shows changes in location (diaphragmatic hernias or ruptures), size (hepatomegaly or microhepatia), echostructure and echogenicity.

DIFFUSE LIVER DISEASES

Diffuse liver diseases can cause general organ deterioration, which affects its size and echogenicity.

The echogenicity can be evaluated by comparison with adjacent organs (spleen and kidney); if normal, the evaluation can be done for the same scanning depth and gain settings. Always remember that a normal liver on ultrasonography does not exclude a diffuse liver disease; so, the final diagnosis often requires a liver biopsy. Table 7.1 and Diagram 7.1 help the diagnostic reasoning by taking into account possible differential diagnoses.

TABLE 7.1
Differential diagnosis for diffuse liver diseases

	Hepatomegaly	From normal size to microhepatia
Hyperechoic liver (Fig. 7.5)	Lipidosis/steatosis Diabetes Steroid liver disease Lymphoma Mast cell tumour	Fibrosis/cirrhosis
Hypoechoic liver (Fig. 7.6)	Congestion Hepatitis/cholangiohepatitis Leukaemias/lymphoma Histiocytic neoplasia	
Heterogeneous liver (Fig. 7.7)	Active chronic hepatitis Hepatocutaneous syndrome (dog) Neoplasm Amyloidosis	Chronic hepatitis

METABOLIC DISEASES (Fig. 7.5)
Lipidosis/steatosis, diabetes mellitus and steroid liver disease cause vacuolar liver disease presenting with:

- Hepatomegaly
- Diffusely hyperechoic or heterogeneous parenchyma (if associated with nodular hyperplasia). Parenchyma echogenicity is higher compared to the adjacent adipose tissue and the spleen; hyperechoic interfaces associated with portal vessels are hardly identifiable
- Increased echoes absorption in distal portions: this produces a hypoechoic appearance of the organ distal part which can not be compensated by increasing the gain
- In these cases, laboratory findings and the ultrasonographic study of adrenal glands are crucial to move towards a diagnosis (hyperglycemia, adrenal hyperplasia and suspected hyperadrenocorticism).

Hepatic amyloidosis is a rare condition except in genetically predisposed individuals (Shar-Pei dogs, Siamese and Oriental breeds cats); the ultrasonographic findings include:

- Hepatomegaly
- Hyperechoic or heterogeneous liver with hypoechoic or hyperechoic liver nodules
- To obtain a diagnosis, other liver diseases must be excluded and any breed predisposition considered. The confirmation is by histopathology.

VENOUS LIVER CONGESTION (Fig. 7.6a)
It is caused by right heart diseases (among the most common, tricuspidal insufficiency, cardiac tamponade due to pericardial effusion) or the compression/obstruction of the caudal vena cava cranially to the diaphragm.

Ultrasonographic findings include:

- Hepatomegaly
- Diffusely hypoechoic parenchyma
- Marked retrograde flow in the Pulsed Wave (PW) Doppler trace line, which becomes positive. Intrahepatic venous branches become more visible and their diameter is greater compared to corresponding portal vessels

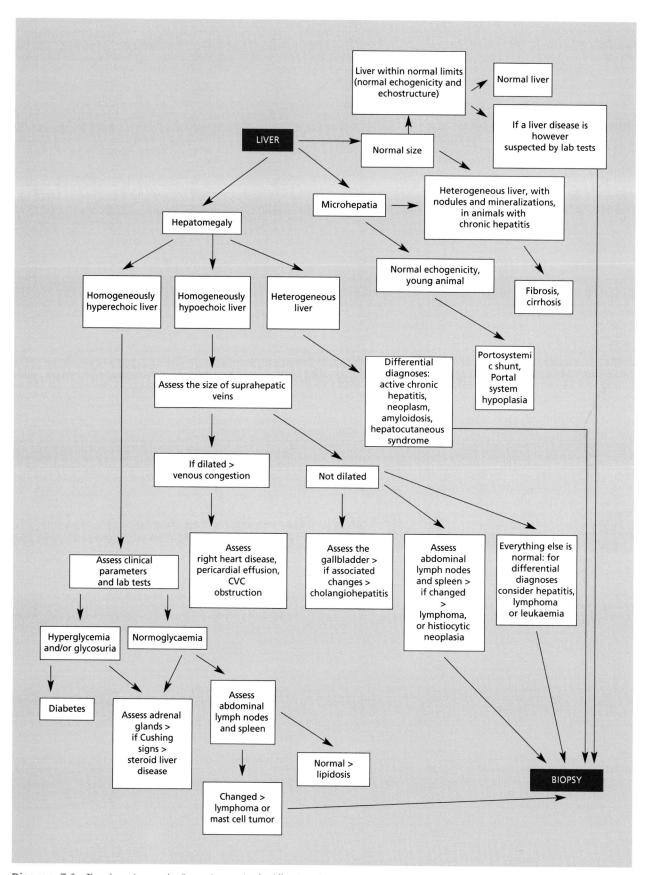

Diagram 7.1   The schematic eases the diagnostic reasoning for diffuse liver changes.

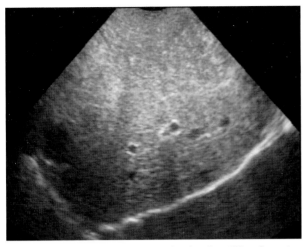

Figure 7.5a Hepatomegaly and hyperechoic liver (steroid liver disease in a dog). Liver echogenicity is similar to adjacent adipose tissue and attenuated distal echoes are visible.

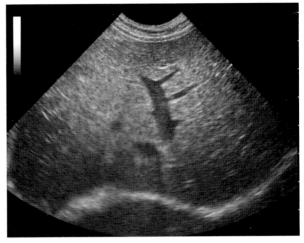

Figure 7.6a Hepatomegaly and hypoechoic liver (liver congestion). Note the suprahepatic veins distension.

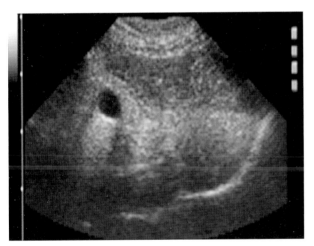

Figure 7.5b Hepatomegaly and hyperechoic liver (diabetes mellitus in a cat). The liver is hyperechoic compared to adipose tissue of the adjacent falciform ligament.

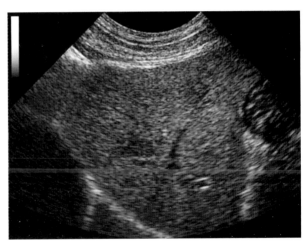

Figure 7.6b Hepatomegaly, hypoechoic liver with some hypoechoic nodules (acute hepatitis). Hypoechoic injuries proved to be liver abscesses (cytological examination).

- Possible associated ascites
- A thoracic cavity ultrasonographic examination is suggested to assess the possible pericardial effusion, right cardiomegaly or obstructive injuries of the caudal vena cava.

HEPATITIS (Fig. 7.6b and 7.7)

Hepatitis or **acute** cholangiohepatitis (Fig. 7.6b) causes:

- Hepatomegaly
- Diffusely hypoechoic liver with increased visibility of hyperechoic periportal tissue. Sometimes, ultrasonographic changes are mild and unrelated to clinical and lab changes, which are often severe. In such cases, a simple needle aspirate is the easiest way to confirm a suspect of hepatitis
- If there are haemorrhages, oedema areas or intrahepatic abscesses, the parenchyma may take a more heterogeneous appearance, with possible focal injuries. In these cases, the ultrasonographic picture is comparable to a liver neoplasm (for example, lymphoma)

- Gallbladder associated changes (sediment, stones, wall thickening)
- Hepatic lymphadenopathy.

Chronic hepatitis (Fig. 7.7) is rather characterized by:

- Normal/small liver
- Hyperechoic parenchyma (secondary to fibrosis) or heterogeneous parenchyma with mineralizations
- Irregular edges, with possible nodules (hyperplasia or nodules associated to cirrhosis)
- Ascites (secondary to portal hypertension or hypoalbuminemia)
- More rarely, lymphadenopathy
- Even chronic forms may show cystic, haemorrhage or necrosis areas at the same time
- In severe cases, with very heterogeneous liver and nodules, differentiating chronic inflammatory process from neoplasm is more difficult. The most important ultrasonographic finding is the liver size, which is normal/reduced in liver cirrhosis and increased in liver neoplasm.

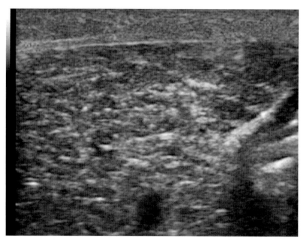

Figure 7.7a Hyperechoic liver with poor visualization of portal vessels (chronic hepatitis and fibrosis). In the caudal edge of the liver lobe, some hypoechoic nodules are visible that make the surface irregular.

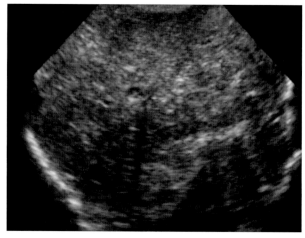

Figure 7.7c Small and hyperechoic liver parenchyma with parenchima mineralizations (chronic hepatitis).

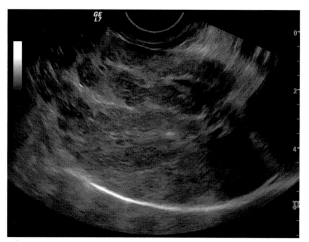

Figure 7.7b Liver cirrhosis. The liver appears hyperechoic and very heterogeneous, fully stuffed with nodules.

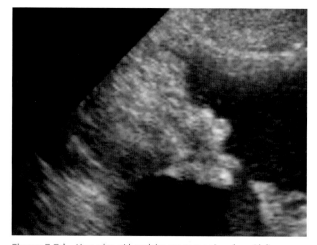

Figure 7.7d Liver edge with nodular appearance in a dog with liver cirrhosis and effusion.

LYMPHOMA (Fig. 7.8)

The literature reports 4 different types of ultrasonographic patterns associated to liver lymphoma:

- Hepatomegaly and normal echogenicity
- Hepatomegaly and diffusely hypoechoic liver
- Hepatomegaly and hypoechoic liver nodules: the most characteristic pattern

- Hepatomegaly and hyperechoic parenchyma: less common.

With suspected liver lymphoma, regional lymph nodes (liver) and all other abdominal organs possibly involved in forms of multicentric lymphoma (visceral lymph nodes, spleen, intestines) must be deeply investigated.

There is often serious lymphadenopathy and multi-organ involvement, which orient towards a diagnosis of lymphoma.

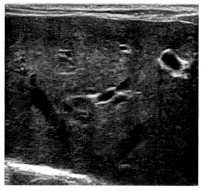

Figure 7.8a Hepatomegaly and hypoechoic liver with hypoechoic nodular injuries (liver lymphoma in a cat).

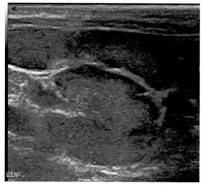

Figure 7.8b Enlarged mesenteric lymph nodes in the same cat.

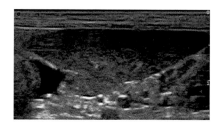

Figure 7.8c Splenomegaly in the same cat. Abdominal effusion is visible as well.

OTHER DIFFUSE LIVER NEOPLASMS

Mast cell tumour, histiocytic sarcoma, and carcinoma can cause liver diffuse infiltration, with hepatomegaly and changes in echogenicity:

- Mast cell tumour: basically hyperechoic parenchyma
- Histiocytic sarcoma: hypoechoic parenchyma, and/or nodules or hypoechoic masses. Often associated with splenic, kidney and lung injuries; moreover, the lymph node involvement is serious
- Carcinoma: mixed echogenicity.

FOCAL LIVER INJURIES

They are a common finding, especially in the elderly. Often benign, so this finding does not necessarily mean a serious liver disease. Even if ultrasonographic findings may suggest the nature of the injury, the ultrasonography specificity in differentiating various focal injuries is low. Therefore, the final diagnosis needs an injury biopsy.

LIVER CYSTS (Fig. 7.9)

Single or multiple, may be congenital, traumatic, inflammatory, parasitic or biliary; often, they are accidental findings without any clinical significance. However, they may be part of benign or malignant (cystadenoma or cystadenocarcinoma) larger injuries. It is therefore important to carefully examine the surrounding liver parenchyma, which in these cases is not normal. In cats, liver cysts can be associated with renal or pericardial cysts as part of a polycystic disease.

On ultrasonography liver cysts appear as:

- Well delimited structures with thin wall
- Anechoic content, rounded, oval or multilobular appearance. The content can become more echoic (corpuscular) with associated haemorrhage or when cysts have a parasitic nature (hydatidosis)
- Posterior-wall enhancement visible.

HAEMATOMA

The haematoma ultrasonographic appearance is variable and changes with the age of injury:

- Acute haemorrhage has a hyperechoic appearance
- Then, the haematoma appears hypoechoic or anechoic
- When clots are reorganized, some of the content can become hyperechoic, giving a heterogeneous appearance to the injury
- After weeks or months, clots can be lysed and their contents anechoic again
- Injury edges are usually irregular and ill-defined.

Often, differentiating a haematoma from another focal injury (abscess, necrosis, neoplasm) is difficult, so the ultrasonographic follow-up can be very useful.

In addition, ultrasonographic findings must be combined with clinical and lab data.

INFARCTION (Fig. 7.10)

Liver infarctions may result from thromboembolism or lobes torsion. The ultrasonographic appearance varies depending on the time between the event and the ultrasonographic

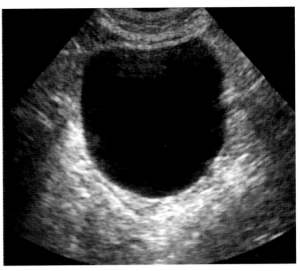

Figure 7.9a   Huge single liver cyst (do not confuse it with the gallbladder).

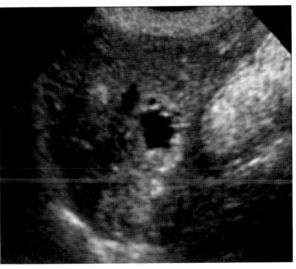

Figure 7.9b   Liver cysts in a feline heterogeneous liver (final diagnosis of cystadenoma).

examination, and the presence of associated injuries (haemorrhage, calcifications). The ultrasonographic appearance of acute infarction is as follows:

- Peripheral location
- Clean edges
- Hypoechoic appearance
- No Doppler stream.

ABSCESS

The ultrasonographic appearance is variable

- Often, injuries are isoechoic or hypoechoic
- Often, they have a central cavitary part containing anechoic or corpuscular material
- Sometimes, they look hypoechoic or mixed (complex mass)
- Edges are regular or irregular
- If gas is present, echoes are associated with reverberations
- Lymphadenomegaly and signs of peritonitis (adjacent hyperechoic peritoneum, effusion) are often associated.

The ultrasonography is very useful to aspirate samples for cytological examination and culture.

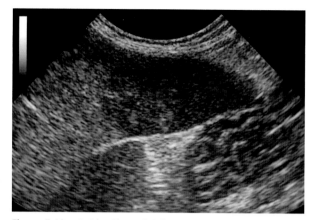

Figure 7.10 Peripheral hypoechoic liver injury with clean edges (infarction).

NODULAR HYPERPLASIA (Fig. 7.11)

Hyperplastic liver nodules are very common in older animals. The most common ultrasonographic appearance features hypoechoic small injuries (<1 cm); however, larger injuries are regularly observed, with variable echogenicity (hypoechoic, iso-echoic, moderately hyperechoic or complex). In these cases, the differential diagnosis with other benign or malignant injuries is impossible and an injury biopsy is needed.

NEOPLASM (Fig. 7.12)

Metastases are more common than primary liver tumours; they spread via the bloodstream (portal vein or hepatic artery), the lymphstream, or by contiguity, and originate from malignant neoplasms of various organs (e.g. gastric, intestinal, pancreatic, and breast carcinoma, spleen sarcomas and lymphosarcoma). They appear as parenchymal nodules.

With a primary neoplasm, a localized mass can be visible; as an alternative, the liver shows increased volume, irregular appearance, single or multiple focal injuries, and changes in the lobar and vascular architecture. Huge liver masses may extend caudally in the abdomen, especially if pedicled, and their origin can be sometimes difficult to establish with certainty. The best way to confirm the hepatic origin is to identify the link with the liver following mass vessels or the vessels of the adjacent parenchyma portion. There are no specific ultrasonographic features for the type of liver primary or metastatic neoplasm, but some patterns are more often associated with some pictures:

- Metastases: the so-called 'target injuries', which appear as hypoechoic nodules with hyperechoic centre, raise a high suspicion of metastases. In the diagnosis of metastases, the literature reports a positive predictive value of 72 per cent for hepatic and splenic target lesions (Cuccovillo et al. 2002)
- Lymphosarcoma and histiocytic sarcoma: they often cause hepatomegaly with hypoechoic liver and hypoechoic nodules/masses, with associated severe lymphadenomegaly
- Hepatocellular carcinoma: it can occur as single injury with hyperechoic or complex appearance, or as multifocal injuries with mixed echogenicity
- Cystadenoma/cystadenocarcinoma: they are characterized by focal or multifocal injuries with a cystic component.

GALLBLADDER AND BILIARY TRACT

BILIARY SLUDGE (Fig.7.13)

It is a suspension of more or less viscous solid/semi-solid particles, that appears on ultrasonography as a hyperechoic sediment in the more declivous portion of the gallbladder and does not produce shadowing. It is a frequent and regular finding in elderly patients and has no clinical significance, especially in dogs. Sometimes, the sludge can get organized to form rounded solid agglomerates (sludge balls).

GALLSTONES (Fig. 7.14)

Not common, they are stones made of cholesterol or salts of bile acids associated with clumps of bile pigments, proteins, fatty acids and phospholipids. They appear as hyperechoic structures with a shape that can be rounded, more irregular (if located in the gallbladder) or linear (if located in bile ducts); they have clean edges and produce shadowing. With stones, the cholecystitis is common, especially in cats. Signs of biliary obstruction are a possible finding.

CHOLECYSTITIS (Fig. 7.14 and 7.15)

It is often associated to hepatitis, and ultrasonographic findings include:

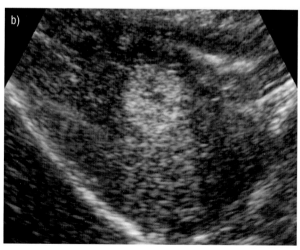

Figure 7.11 Examples of liver nodular hyperplasia with hypoechoic **(a)** and hyperechoic **(b)** appearance.

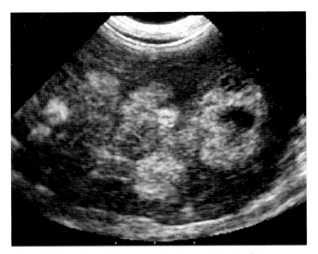

Figure 7.12a Huge heterogeneous hepatic mass (hepatocellular carcinoma).

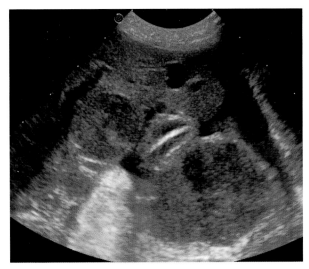

Figure 7.12c Multiple liver nodules, which change the hepatic architecture (metastases). There is also an anechoic abdominal effusion.

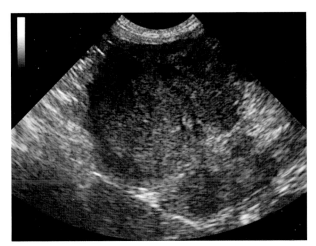

Figure 7.12b Hypoechoic liver mass (liver adenoma).

If gas is present (emphysematous cholecystitis) there are hyperechoic foci that follow organ edges and produce reverberation artefacts; in these cases an accurate wall evaluation is very important to exclude any discontinuities that could indicate necrosis and rupture, a relatively common occurrence with serious infections
- Chronic cholecystitis: wall thickening and irregularities, hyperechoic appearance, possible areas of mineralization. The gallbladder fibrosis may prevent the organ distension, so it appears very small
- The inner surface of the wall (which corresponds to the mucous coat) is irregular
- Changes of biliary content (increased echogenicity, stones)
- Thickening or dilation of the common bile duct (secondary to inflammation or obstruction due to inflammatory material in the biliary tract) is often associated.

Often, the gallbladder compression due to the ultrasonographic probe is painful.

Note that the gallbladder wall oedema may also occur with

- Acute cholecystitis: diffuse thickening of the gallbladder wall, with possible double-walled appearance caused by inflammatory oedema; it shows two hyperechoic interfaces separated by an intermediate hypoechoic layer.

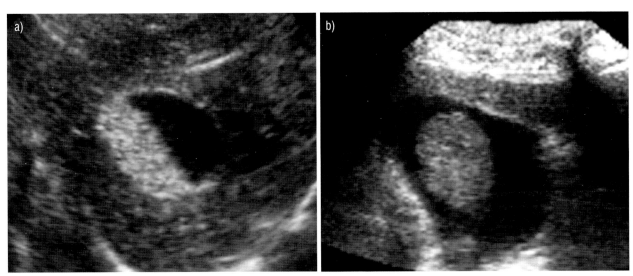

Figure 7.13 Biliary sludge that settles in the gallbladder declivous portion **(a)** or tends to form an oval agglutinate **(b)**.

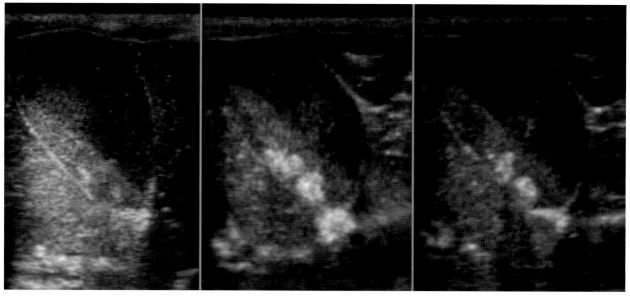

Figure 7.14 Cholecystitis and gallstones. The gallbladder wall is thickened, there are abundant sediments and stones that generate shadowing.

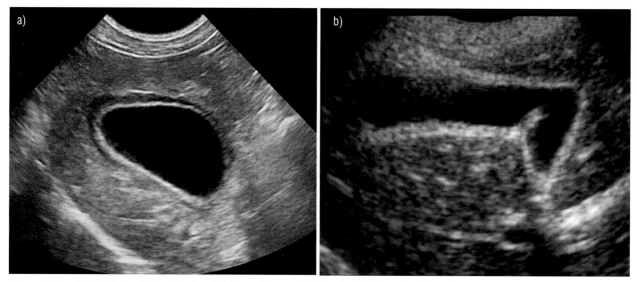

Figure 7.15 **a)** Acute cholecystitis in a dog: the gallbladder wall is strongly thickened, with thickened and hyperechoic mucous coat and double-walled appearance. **b)** Chronic cholecystitis in a cat: the gallbladder is small, the wall is thickened and hyperechoic.

non-inflammatory causes (hypoalbuminemia, portal hypertension, biliary obstruction).

MUCOCELE (Fig. 7.16)

A pathological condition characterized by biliary stasis associated with hyperplasia of the gallbladder mucous coat.

It may be an incidental finding in asymptomatic animals, but is often associated with a bacterial infection of the biliary tract; it may cause the rupture of the wall of the gallbladder, resulting in peritoneal migration of the mucocele and biliary peritonitis (surgical emergency).

On ultrasonography you see:

- Severe gallbladder distension
- Changes of the gallbladder wall (thickening, irregularities)
- Hyperechoic content with starry or finely striated appearance, which generally occupies the whole organ, and is motionless. Appearance similar to a kiwi slice
- Possible discontinuities of the gallbladder wall: they are

difficult to visualize with certainty, also due to clots, fibrin and sediment that settle on the wall. In case of rupture, the gallbladder may lose its oval shape
- Effusion adjacent to the gallbladder (in case of wall rupture): carefully examine peritoneum areas adjacent to the gallbladder, searching also for small anechoic layers that may indicate an effusion.Biliary Obstruction (Fig. 7.17 And 7.18)

BILIARY OBSTRUCTION (Fig. 7.17 and 7.18)

The ultrasonographic examination is useful to identify the obstruction cause, which can be intraluminal (stones, neoplasms, parasites), intramural (inflammatory processes or neoplasms) or extramural (pancreas, liver, duodenum, or lymph nodes inflammatory or neoplastic injuries).

The ultrasonographic appearance of the biliary obstruction varies with time:

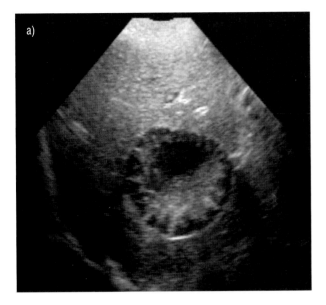

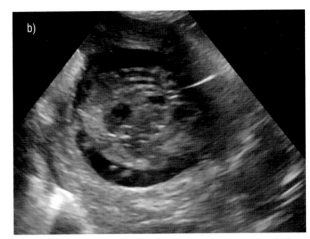

Figure 7.16   **a)** Mucocele in a dog, transverse scan. Typical 'kiwi slice' appearance with fine stripes arranged in a radial pattern and directed from the centre to the periphery. **b)** Mucocele, longitudinal scan. In this case, the mucocele is a heterogeneous mass that occupies all the gallbladder lumen. Note the severe wall thickening and hypoechogenicity.

- First 24 hours: the gallbladder and the cystic duct dilate
- After 48 hours: dilation of the common bile duct (diameter >4 mm in cats) with tortuous appearance
- After 5–7 days: in case of complete obstruction, dilatation of lobar ducts. Intrahepatic bile ducts appear as intrahepatic

tubular structures with a tortuous course that can be distinguished from vessels as they are not branches of great vessels (portal vein or caudal vena cava) and do not show a flow on the Doppler examination.

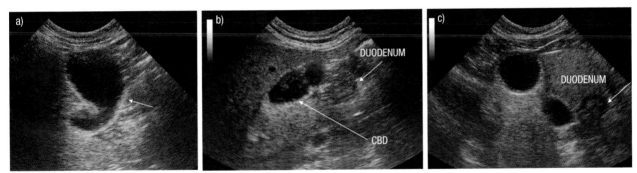

Figure 7.17   A cat with cholangiohepatitis and biliary obstruction. Note the gallbladder wall thickening **(a)**, and the CBD dilatation which continues up to its entry into the duodenum **(b and c)**.

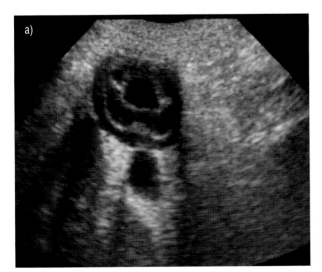

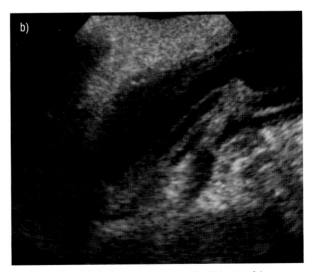

Figure 7.18   A dog with chronic pancreatitis, duodenitis, and CBD obstruction. Note the hyperechogenicity in the pancreatic region, the thickening of the duodenal wall and the distension of the last CBD tract, which is thickened and hyperechoic at the duodenal papilla.

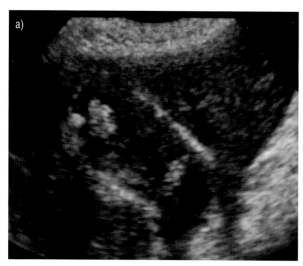
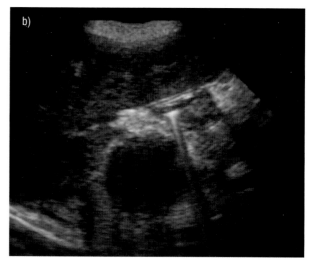

Figure 7.19   Two examples of biliary tract carcinoma arising from the gallbladder **(a)** and the common bile duct **(b)**. **a)** The gallbladder has a broken wall and is occupied by a partially mineralized mass. **b)** In the region between the liver, the duodenum and the pancreas, an ill-defined hypoechoic injury extends cranially to the liver and infiltrates the surrounding peritoneum.

Moreover, thickening, foreign material (sludge, stones) or masses affecting the common bile duct are associated.

Even if the obstruction is resolved, the biliary tract dilatation may remain.

NEOPLASMS (Fig. 7.19)
Polyps and malignant neoplasms of the biliary tract are relatively infrequent.

- Polyps appear as rounded pedicled injuries protruding into the gallbladder lumen
- Malignant neoplasms cause loss of wall definition, and generate masses involving the adjacent liver, the biliary tract and other adjacent structures (peritoneum, pancreas, lymph nodes).

RECOMMENDED READING

Lamb CR, Hartzband LE, Tidwell AS, Pearson SH: Ultrasonographic findings in hepatic and splenic lymphosarcoma in dogs and cats. Vet Rad 1991; 32: 117–120.

Stowater et al. Ultrasonographic features of canine hepatic nodular hyperplasia. Vet Radiol & Ultrasound 1990; 31(5): 268–272.

Newell SM et al.: Correlations between ultrasonographic findings and specific hepatic diseases in cats: 72 cases (1985–1997) JAVMA 1998; 213(1): 94–98.

Schwarz LA et al. Hepatic abscesses in 13 dogs: a review of the ultrasonographic findings, clinical data and therapeutic options. Vet Radiol & Ultrasound 1998; 39(4): 357–365.

Nyland T. et al. Ultrasonographic evaluation of biliary cystadenomas in cats. Vet Radiol & Ultrasound 1999; 40(3): 300–306.

Besso JG et al. Ultrasonographic appearance and clinical findings in 14 dogs with gallbladder mucocele. Vet Radiol & Ultrasound 2000; 41(3): 261–271.

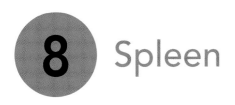

8 Spleen

Gian Marco Gerboni

SCAN TECHNIQUE (FIG. 8.1–6)

Animal preparation	• 12 hours on an empty stomach, at least. • Wide hair-clipping, including the last left intercostal spaces. • Dorsal recumbency, right lateral.
Probes	• Microconvex, 7.5 MHz mean frequency in dogs and 10 MHz mean frequency in cats (5–10 MHz in case of splenomegaly). • Linear high-frequency (7.5–10 MHz) for small breed animals and organ surface portions.
Scans and respective probe position	Positions for the spleen scan are partly variables since the only fixed portion of the organ is the head; in contrast, body and tail move according to their size, the gastric repletion and the position of the other abdominal organs. The scan must be therefore adapted to these variables, following the spleen in the middle abdomen and possibly the caudal abdomen. It is important to make sure to visualize the whole organ, including the most dorsal portion of the head located below the costal arch, so as to not miss important parts and possible injuries. • **Longitudinal scan** (position 5 to 11, Fig. 8.2): with the probe perpendicular to the skin surface, start from the left cranial abdomen, a bit ventrally to the costal arch, where a portion of the organ body is identified. The probe is aligned to the spleen long axis, then moved in the caudoventral direction following the body and the tail. • **Transverse scan** (position 5 to 11, Fig. 8.3): with the probe perpendicular to the skin surface, from the longitudinal scan rotate the probe by 90° and follow the organ that appears triangular in shape, from the head to the tail. • **Intercostal scans** (position 5 to 6): the probe is perpendicular to the skin surface, over the last two left intercostal spaces. The probe is aligned parallel to the ribs, then rotated in the transverse plane. The splenic head, triangular in shape and located between gastric fundus and left kidney, is visualized.

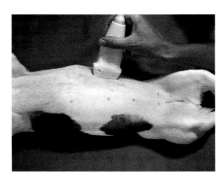

Figure 8.1a Position 5. Spleen longitudinal scan. Linear probe.

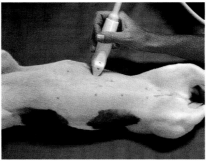

Figure 8.1b Position 5. Spleen transverse scan. Linear probe.

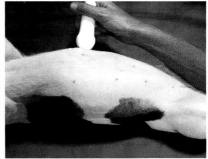

Figure 8.1c Left intercostal scan, searching for the splenic head. From position 5, the probe is moved dorsally over the last 2 intercostal spaces, to position 6. Microconvex probe.

ULTRASONOGRAPHIC ANATOMY (Fig. 8.2–6)

Location	• Left and middle cranial abdomen.
Morphology	**Linguiform**, it has 2 sides: a convex parietal aspect and a concave visceral aspect where vascular structures enter at the hilum level. The organ is composed of: • **Head** (Fig. 8.3): lies cranially, between the gastric fundus and the diaphragm. • **Body** (Fig. 8.4): parallel to the gastric curvature. • **Tail**: runs along the left abdominal wall in the caudal direction; very mobile, it also moves to the right of median plan in the middle and caudal abdomen. **NB**: sometimes an island of splenic parenchyma separated from the organ (accessory spleen) is visible and located in perisplenic fat (Fig. 8.4). **NB**: sometimes nodular hyperechogenicity areas are visible on the mesenteric side, associated with the first part of splenic veins (see also Focal injuries – myelolipomas) (Fig. 8.5).
Relationships with adjacent organs evaluable on ultrasonography	• **Head**: cranially to the fundus of the stomach, caudally and medially to the cranial pole of the left kidney, laterally to the left abdominal wall. • **Body**: medially to the stomach, laterally to left kidney and left abdominal wall. Variable relationship with loops of small intestine and large intestine. • **Tail**: variable relationship with the organs in the middle abdomen; caudally it can reach the bladder cranial pole.
Size	**Subjective evaluation**: some parameters are to be considered • Thickness. • Position of the ventral end (folded tail). • Shape of edges (in case of splenomegaly, edges are rounded).
Edges	• Thin, smooth and regular.
Echogenicity	• Medium/high. • Hypoechoic parenchyma compared to the adipose tissue and the prostate. • Hyperechoic parenchyma compared to the renal cortex and the liver. • Thin hyperechoic capsule only visible in areas where the ultrasound beam is perfectly perpendicular.
Echostructure	• Homogeneous. • Finely granular and more homogeneous compared to the liver echostructure.
Vessels (Fig. 8.8 and 8.9)	**Splenic vein** (Fig. 8.8) • Anechoic tubular structure with straight course, parallel to the organ longitudinal axis, it receives several branches (2–5 dorsally and 4–9 ventrally). • It can be followed from the splenic hilum in the cranial direction; it turns medially to end in the portal vein. The last tract is an important landmark to locate the pancreas left lobe, which is in contact with the confluence of this vessel into the portal vein. • Easily compressible lumen. **Branches of the splenic v.:** • Anechoic tubular structures that penetrate the visceral surface along the hilum, have a 'Y' shape and thin wall that is not normally visible. • Diameter similar to hepatic veins, they get thinner and less and less visible proceeding into the parenchyma. **NB**: in some patients, the splenic veins' flow is slow enough to allow the visualization of echoic endoluminal movable content, particularly in sedated patients and using a high-frequency probe. This must not be considered a clear pathological situation (for example, predisposition to thromboembolism). It is also found in dogs with autoimmune anaemia (Fig. 8.9). Splenic artery: can be identified using the Doppler function; it comes from the celiac artery and runs parallel with venous structures.
Tributary lymph nodes	**Splenic**

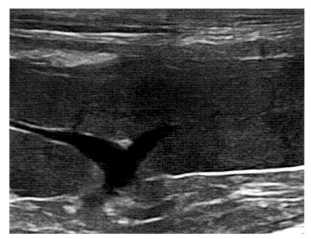

Figure 8.2 Longitudinal scan of a normal spleen. The image shows part of the body and the hilum with a splenic vein branch. Distinctive "Y" appearance of splenic vein branches within the parenchyma. Veins are the only normally visible vascular structures within the parenchyma.

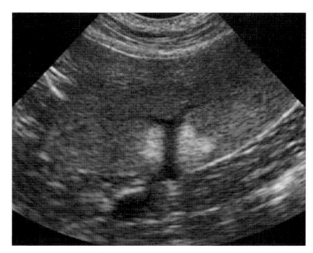

Figure 8.5 Normal spleen with marked hyperechogenicity located where the branch enters the splenic vein. This non-pathological change is created by the perivascular intussusception of the hilar fat and the capsule. Some authors also call this finding myelolipoma.

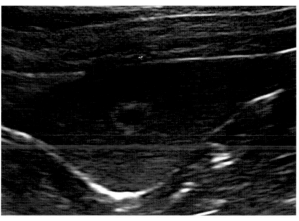

Figure 8.3 Normal spleen (head) in the transverse scan obtained with the dog in dorsal recumbency; the thin and echoic capsule is well visible where echoes intersect it perpendicularly.

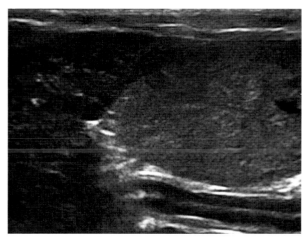

Figure 8.6 Spleen normal echogenicity. Comparison of echogenicity and echostructure between the splenic parenchyma and the liver parenchyma. Note that the spleen parenchyma echogenicity is higher compared to the liver, while the spleen echostructure is finer than the liver one.

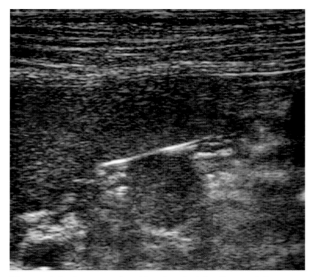

Figure 8.4 Accessory spleen. Near the splenic head, a rounded structure surrounded by peritoneal fat is visible, whose echogenicity and echostructure are very similar to the splenic parenchyma.

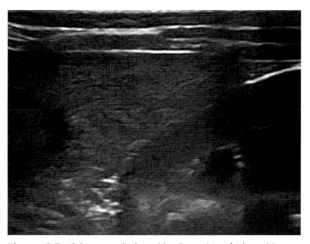

Figure 8.7 Spleen normal echogenicity. Comparison of echogenicity between the splenic parenchyma and the renal cortex. Note that the echogenicity of the splenic parenchyma is higher.

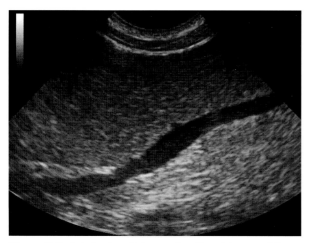

Figure 8.8 Splenic vein and intraparenchymal branch in a normal dog. The vessel lumen appears anechoic.

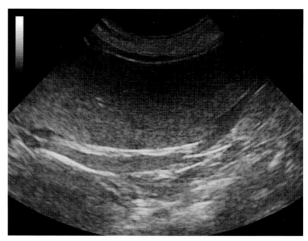

Figure 8.9 Spleen and splenic vein of a dog with autoimmune haemolytic anaemia. There is a marked echogenicity of the vessel lumen secondary to red blood cells autoagglutination.

ULTRASONOGRAPHIC CHANGES

SPLENOMEGALY (Fig. 8.10)
All infiltrative diseases (inflammatory or neoplastic) show a general increase in the organ volume; the increase in spleen volume involves the following ultrasonographic findings:

- Increase in organ thickness and length
- The spleen extends caudally to reach the cranial edge of the bladder
- The caudal portion folds back on itself
- Edges become rounded.

REDUCTION IN SPLEEN SIZE (Fig. 8.11)
It happens when the blood reserve contained in the splenic pulp is used, mainly due to severe haemorrhage or shock. The spleen appears smaller than normal, almost completely housed under the costal arch, while the parenchyma echogenicity and echostructure are normal.

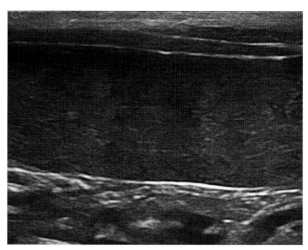

Figure 8.10 Splenomegaly. The passive congestion can also increase the spleen thickness.

SPLEEN DIFFUSE CHANGES

Table 8.1 summarizes the main changes in spleen echogenicity and echostructure.
The spleen venous congestion creates aspecific changes.
Acute congestion creates:

- Splenomegaly, visible as increased body thickness, and rounded edges
- Diffuse reduction in echogenicity
- Enlargement of splenic veins and their branches without parenchyma changes.

The protracted congestion becomes **chronic** and causes:

- Increased volume
- Diffused increase in the parenchyma echogenicity
- Enlargement of splenic veins and branches more visible within the parenchyma
- Irregular edges.

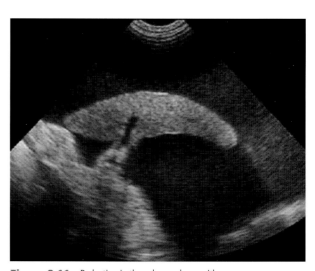

Figure 8.11 Reduction in the spleen volume with severe haemoabdomen. The parenchyma appears normoechoic and homogeneous (within normal limits).

TABLE 8.1 Major changes in spleen echogenicity and echostructure		
	Single or multiple parenchyma focal injuries	Parenchyma diffuse injuries
Isoechoic homogeneous	Nodular hyperplasia	Passive congestion Torsion Lymphosarcoma Splenic hyperplasia
Hypoechoic homogeneous	Nodular hyperplasia Extramedullary haematopoiesis Metastases Haemangioma Lymphosarcoma Mast cell tumour Acute inflammation (splenitis) Haematoma Infarction - necrosis Abscesses Cysts More rarely, haemangiosarcoma	Passive congestion Splenic torsion Lymphosarcoma Mast cell tumour Acute inflammation
Hyperechoic homogeneous	Myelolipomas Recent haematoma Fibrosis Parasitic granulomas More rarely, metastases	Chronic passive congestion Mast cell tumour Chronic inflammation (splenitis) Senile atrophy
Heterogeneous or mixed	Haemangiosarcoma, typical appearance Haemangioma Lymphosarcoma Metastases Haematoma Infarction – necrosis More rarely, nodular hyperplasia	

Spleen changes must be evaluated taking into account modifications of portal vein, caudal vena cava and hepatic veins. The passive congestion is often secondary to portal hypertension, or pressure changes of the caudal vena cava.

SPLEEN TORSION (Fig. 8.12)

The spleen ultrasonographic appearance varies as a function of time length and torsion degree.

In a recent torsion, changes are similar to those of passive congestion.

In case of persistent torsion, the spleen shows:

- Clear increase in volume and rounded edges
- Reduction in parenchyma echogenicity

- A 'tubular' appearance of the parenchyma created by severe congestion of vessels and sinusoids that appear as thin anechoic structures arranged in parallel and separated by hyperechoic lines that correspond to vessel walls. This typical pattern is described in English as 'lace-like', since its appearance resembles a lace
- Splenic veins and vascular pedicles show a strongly hyperechoic triangular shape, with distal echoes dispersion localized in the hilum and in continuity with the mesentery. The lumen of venous structures is not visible
- Associated changes: thrombosis of splenic vein proximal branches.

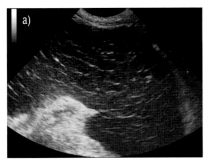 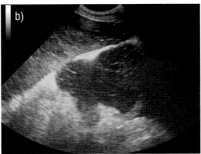 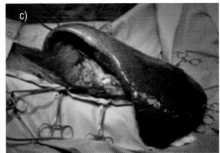

Figure 8.12 Spleen torsion. a) The spleen is increased in volume, hypoechoic, with parenchyma tubular echostructure (highlighted by parallel echoic lines); the usual course of splenic veins branches cannot be followed. b) The spleen is hypoechoic compared to the liver parenchyma; branches of splenic veins are often thrombosed and the echogenicity in the hilar region increased. c) Intraoperative finding.

The vascular Doppler eases the diagnosis of torsion. The differential diagnosis between torsion and splenomegaly associated with vascular changes (thromboembolism, splenic infarctions) may be difficult; studying the splenic vessels flow, special attention must be paid to the position of spleen portions, the hilum appearance (presence or absence of hyperechoic triangular structure) and possible Colour Doppler abnormalities.

ACUTE AND CHRONIC SPLENITIS (Fig. 8.13–14)

A number of situations can activate the spleen; among these, systemic infectious diseases with bacterial and fungal origin, primary spleen infections or autoimmune diseases.

The ultrasonographic appearance of **acute** forms is characterized by:

- Normal/increased size
- Decreased echogenicity
- Changes associated with the inflammation and necrosis degree (thrombosis, infarction and abscess).

The **chronic** splenitis instead is characterized by:

- Normal/increased size

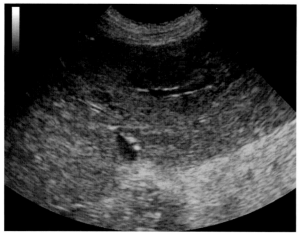

Figure 8.13 Chronic splenitis. The size is often normal with increased echogenicity, non-uniform echostructure and irregular edges, non-stretched venous branches.

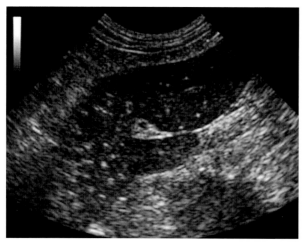

Figure 8.14 Spleen diffuse mineralizations. Non-uniform echostructure due to hyperechoic dot-like multifocal injuries, that are the outcome of a chronic splenitis.

- Increased echogenicity
- Intraparenchymal calcification foci
- Changed edges (irregular).

DIFFUSE NEOPLASTIC DISEASES

The most common neoplasms that cause spleen diffuse infiltration are lymphosarcoma, mast cell tumour, malignant histiocytoma and leukaemias. In cats, the splenomegaly is most often associated with neoplastic diseases, while in the dog aspecific activation conditions prevail. Ultrasonographic changes observed with diffuse neoplasms of the splenic parenchyma are aspecific and include splenomegaly, diffuse changes in increased or decreased echogenicity, heterogeneous appearance. Some of these tumours are, however, more often associated with some findings, which can direct the diagnosis.

LYMPHOSARCOMA (DIFFUSE FORM) (Fig. 8.15)

Note that the splenic lymphosarcoma may present as diffuse form (here described), as nodular form (see below) or a combination of the two.

- Splenomegaly
- Variable echogenicity, diffusely hypoechoic spleen
- Non-dilated splenic veins and branches
- Altered echostructure, with characteristic honeycomb or wax cells appearance
- Associated changes (hypoechoic or anechoic nodules, lymphadenopathy of splenic lymph nodes).

MAST CELL TUMOUR (Fig. 8.16)

- Splenomegaly
- Variable echogenicity, diffusely hypoechoic or hyperechoic spleen
- Non-dilated splenic veins and branches
- Irregular edges and borders.

SPLEEN FOCAL OR MULTIFOCAL CHANGES

This group includes benign and malignant injuries that can have different sizes and a variable and overlapping ultrasonographic

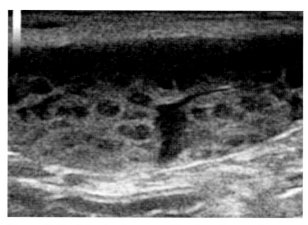

Figure 8.15 Spleen lymphosarcoma, diffuse form. The parenchyma echostructure has a 'wax cells' or 'honeycomb' appearance due to small hypoechoic focal injuries disseminated throughout the parenchyma.

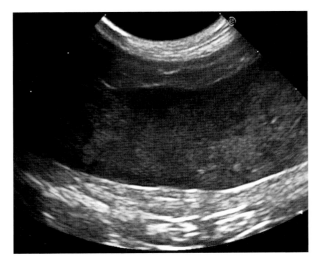

Figure 8.16 Spleen mast cell tumour in a dog. The parenchyma is not homogeneous and there is a marked reduction in echogenicity, especially at a subcapsular level.

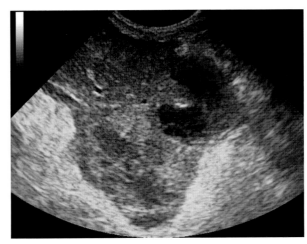

Figure 8.17 Haematoma with an organizing clot. On the left side of the image, the normal parenchyma is visible. In the central portion, the mass echostructure is non-uniform, partly echoic and organized, partly anechoic and cystic. The ultrasonography cannot differentiate a haematoma from a neoplastic injury; only the lesion evolution allows for a definitive diagnosis.

appearance. There is a real difficulty to differentiate these injuries, even if some injury ultrasonographic findings, and the status of lymph nodes and other abdominal organs, help to find the most likely diagnosis. The definitive diagnosis requires a cytologic/histopathologic injury examination.

HAEMATOMA (Fig. 8.17)
The splenic haematoma can be caused by traumas or haemostasis defects, or associated with spleen neoplasms.

- Single, multiple, subcapsular or intraparenchymal
- Edges altered in greater size injuries
- Echogenicity evolves over time, according to the clot reorganization phase after the haemorrhage
  - First 24 hours: iso-hyperechoic
  - 48–96 hours later: hypo-anechoic
  - Over 96 hours later: hyperechoic.

INFARCTION (Fig. 8.18)
Spleen infarction is mainly the complication of systemic diseases (for example, hyperadrenocorticism, immunomediated anaemia, sepsis). The ultrasonographic appearance is variable, and depends on the extent of involved vessel.

If a small vessel is involved: the injury is peripheral and localized, with triangular or rounded shape and the base positioned towards the periphery.

If a larger vessel is involved: there are larger areas with changes in echogenicity, but they are less easily definable.
In both cases:

- The echogenicity is decreased in acute phases
- During resolution, the injury appears hyperechoic, due to reorganization, and a possibly associated fibrosis
- Associated changes: thrombosis in proximal and intraparenchymal branches of the splenic vein, haematomas.

NODULAR HYPERPLASIA (Fig. 8.19)
Common benign change in dogs older than 10 years. Generally, the liver is also affected.

- Single or multiple nodules with variable diameter (generally <20 mm)
- Not delimited by wall or capsule
- Mostly hypoechoic appearance; however, sometimes isoechoic/hyperechoic

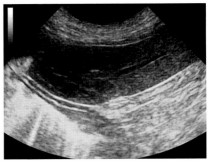

Figure 8.18a Spleen infarction. Acute injury (24 hours): 'rounded' hypoechoic shape localized to the splenic head. Injury edges are linear and rounded.

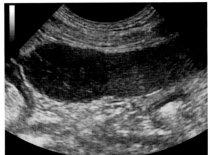

Figure 8.18b Spleen infarction. Check-up after about seven days. Injury size decreased and echogenicity is more similar to the normal parenchyma.

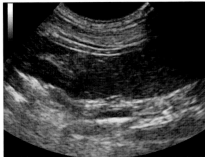

Figure 8.18b Spleen infarction. Check-up after 30 days. The injury is organized. Injury size reduced, the echogenicity is similar to the normal parenchyma and the capsule is regular.

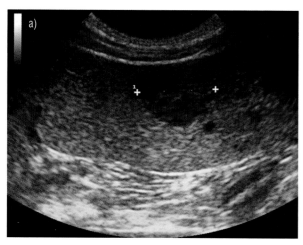

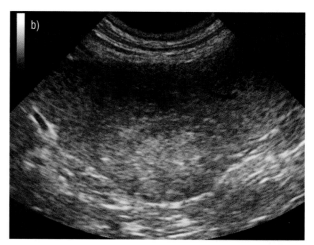

Figure 8.19 Nodular hyperplasia. a) Hypoechoic nodule, well-defined in the parenchyma and delimited by two cursors. b) Hyperechoic nodule with undefined edges, that warps the spleen shape.

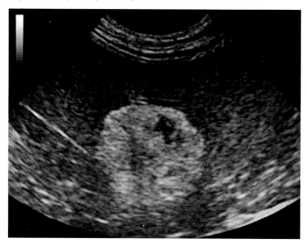

Figure 8.20 Granuloma. Longitudinal scan of the splenic body. Well-defined hyperechoic nodular injury that overflows the capsule. Incidental injury with undetermined aetiology.

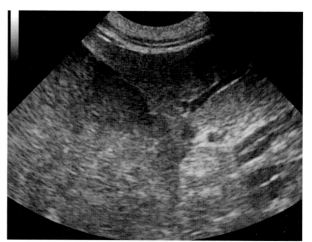

Figure 8.21 Mass in continuity with the splenic body; on the right of the image the normal parenchyma is visible from which the tumour structure originates.

- With peripheral injuries, the splenic edge appears warped and the capsule irregular
- Normally they do not change the splenic vascularization.

ABSCESS/GRANULOMA (Fig. 8.20)
Rare in dogs and cats

- Single or multiple, variably sized injuries
- Echoic wall and little/null posterior-wall enhancement
- Variable echogenicity content, from hypoechoic or corpuscular (abscess), to more echoic (granuloma)
- Suspected abscess in case of reverberation artefacts (gas)
- Irregular edges and/or capsule.

FOCAL OR MULTIFOCAL NEOPLASTIC DISEASES

Spleen focal or multifocal injuries are often caused by sarcomas. Haemangiosarcoma and lymphosarcoma are the most represented. Less common represented are leiomyosarcoma, fibrosarcoma, undifferentiated sarcoma, osteosarcoma, chondrosarcoma, liposarcoma, myxosarcoma, rhabdomyosarcoma and histiocytoma. These neoplasms may present as nodules or masses with variable size, shape and echogenicity (Fig. 8.21).

LYMPHOSARCOMA (NODULAR FORM) (Fig. 8.22)
In dogs, note that the splenic lymphosarcoma may occur in nodular form (described here), diffuse form (described previously), or a combination of the two.

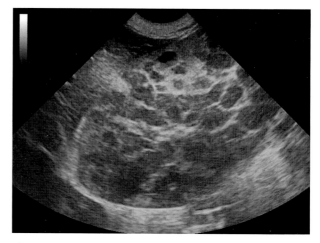

Figure 8.22 Spleen lymphosarcoma, nodular form. Spleen echostructure is heterogeneous, with macular appearance due to rounded hypoechoic focal injuries.

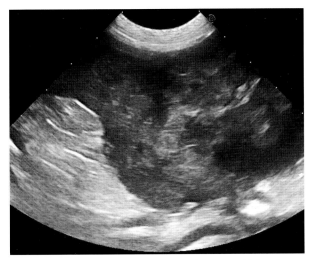

Figure 8.23   Spleen haemangiosarcoma in dogs. Mass with irregular edges, heterogeneous echostructure and cavitary areas with anechoic content.

- Multiple hypoechoic-anechoic nodules with variable sizes
- Not delimited by wall or capsule
- No posterior-wall enhancement
- Warped edges and capsule in larger injuries
- Non-dilated splenic vein and its branches
- Associated injuries (splenomegaly, parenchyma hypoechogenicity, lymphadenopathy of splenic lymph nodes).

HAEMANGIOSARCOMA (Fig. 8.23)
- Complex variably sized injuries (from a nodule to a mass)
- Common portions of normal spleen
- Heterogeneous echostructure with solid or cavitary appearance, and hypoechoic, hyperechoic or anechoic areas (complex mass)
- Posterior-wall enhancement
- Irregular borders and edges
- Non-dilated splenic vein and its branches
- Associated changes (free abdominal fluid; liver, heart and lung metastases).

METASTASES
Metastatic injuries are less common than liver injuries. Similarly to what has already been reported for the liver, the presence of 'target-like' injuries (Fig. 8.24), with hyperechoic centre and anechoic periphery, strongly suggest the metastatic origin of nodules.

THROMBOSIS OF SPLENIC VESSELS (Fig. 8.25)
The thrombosis of splenic veins goes with many spleen diseases that have a vascular, inflammatory and neoplastic origin. The already slow flow of the splanchnic circulation promotes the formation of intravascular thrombi, which appear on ultrasonography as endoluminal motionless hyperechoic foci. The Doppler examination reveals filling defects in these locations. When a thrombus is visualized, surrounding tissues must be carefully evaluated to rule out any masses that infiltrate the vessel. Thrombi can be associated with infarction injuries of the parenchyma.

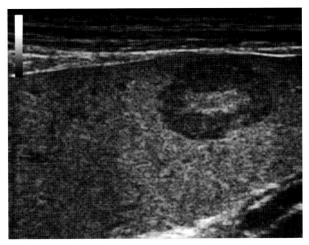

Figure 8.24   Target-like injury. Longitudinal image of a splenic parenchyma which shows a single injury characterized by hyperechoic centre and hypoechoic periphery.

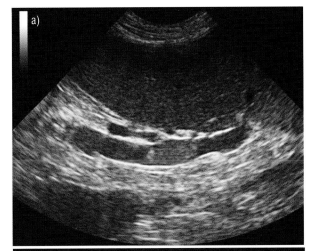

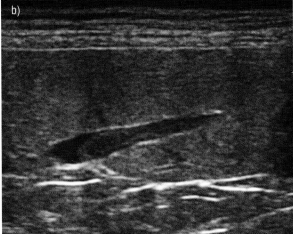

Figure 8.25   Thrombosis of the splenic vein. **a)** The lumen of the splenic vein contains an echoic structure. There are no obvious parenchyma changes. **b)** Thrombosis of an intraparenchymal branch of the splenic vein with no parenchyma infarctions.

RECOMMENDED READING

Sharpley JL, Marolf AJ, Reichle JK, Bachand AM, Randall EK. Color and power Doppler ultrasonography for characterization of splenic masses in dogs. Vet Radiol Ultrasound. 2012, 53: 586–590.

Crabtree AC, Spangler E, Beard D, Smith A. Diagnostic accuracy of gray-scale ultrasonography for the detection of hepatic and splenic lymphoma in dogs. Vet Radiol Ultrasound. 2010, 51: 661–664.

Mai W. The hilar perivenous hyperechoic triangle as a sign of acute splenic torsion in dogs. Vet Radiol Ultrasound. 2006, 47: 487–491.

O'Brien RT, Waller KR, Osgoot TL. Sonographic features of druginduced splenic congestion. Vet Radiol Ultrasound. 2004, 45: 225–227.

Cuccovillo A, Lamb CR. Cellular features of sonographic target lesion of the liver and spleen in 21 dogs and a cat. Vet Radiol Ultrasound. 2002, 43: 275–278.

Hanson JA, Papageorges M, Girard E, Menard M, Hebert P. Ultrasonographic appearance of splenic disease in 101 cat. Vet Radiol Ulrasound. 2001, 42: 441–445.

Schwarz LA, Penninck DG, Gliatto J. Canine splenic myelolipomas. Vet Radiol Ultrasound. 2001, 42: 347–348.

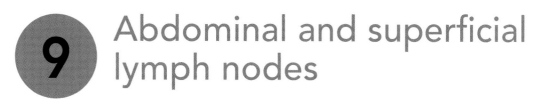

9 Abdominal and superficial lymph nodes

Elvanessa Caleri

Ultrasonography is one of the most sensitive methods to study abdominal lymph nodes, and allows the evaluation of their shape, size, echostructure and echogenicity. Given the small size of lymph nodes and considering that they are often isoechoic compared to surrounding tissues, it is essential to have high-resolution ultrasonographic equipment and good knowledge of landmarks and lymphatic drainage of various organs.

Abdominal lymph nodes that can be explored on ultrasonography can be divided into two groups: visceral lymph nodes and parietal lymph nodes that, in turn, include several lymphocentres. Tables 9.1 and 9.2 and Fig. 9.1 show the abdominal lymph nodes that can be explored on ultrasonography, and the anatomical and ultrasound landmarks useful to locate them.

In addition to abdominal lymph nodes, there are important superficial lymph nodes that can be investigated on

TABLE 9.1 Visceral lymph nodes				
Lymph nodes	Anatomical site	Number and size (length)	Probe position	Ultrasound landmarks
CRANIAL MESENTERIC LYMPHOCENTRE				
Digiunal (or cranial mesenteric)	Root of mesentery of jejunum and ileum, around great mesenteric vessels (artery and vein)	Usually 2; 4–6 cm	Middle abdomen, central position (11)	They are aligned along great vessels of the root of mesentery (mesenteric v. and a.). The initial landmark is the splenic tail; from here the probe is moved searching for great mesenteric vessels and exploring the surrounding mesenteric tissue
Colic	**Right:** ascending colon origin, near the ileocecocolic valve. **Middle:** transverse colon mesentery	Right colic, usually single; the middle may be single or double, 1–2.5 cm	Middle abdomen, slightly to the right of the mid-line (11)	Right: the cecum or the ileocecocolic junction are visualized and the surrounding fat explored. Middle: adjacent to the transverse colon. Often, they are identified in the same image, especially in cats
MESENTERIC CAUDAL LYMPHOCENTRE				
Caudal mesenteric (also called left colic)	Descending mesocolon, near the pelvis	From 2 to 5; 0.5–2 cm	Middle-caudal abdomen, on the left of the mid-line (11)	The descending colon is followed towards the pelvis, then the surrounding mesenteric tissue is explored. They are not visible if unchanged
COELIAC LYMPHOCENTRE				
Gastric	Lesser gastric curvature, near the pylorus	Generally there is only one, but may be missing or double; 0.5–2.5 cm	Cranial abdomen, slightly to the right or sometimes to the left of the mid-line, in contact with the costal arch (start from position 7, then move slightly to position 6 or 8)	The region between the liver and the stomach is explored, along the lesser gastric curvature. More often marked if changed; rarely visible if normal
Pancreaticoduodenal	Lesser curvature of the duodenum, in the omentum and ventrally to the pancreas	They may be missing; 1.5 cm	Cranial abdomen, on the right, in contact with the costal arch (position 8)	When pylorus and descending duodenum are identified, the region caudal to these structures is explored, between them and the pancreas. Identifiable if changed
Hepatic	**Left and right:** 1–2 cm from the porta hepatis, along the portal vein course	2–3 cm	Cranial abdomen, slightly to the right of the mid-line (8)	The landmark is the portal vein, about 1–2 cm caudally to the porta hepatis. Fat tissue is explored, on the left and the right of the portal vein. More identifiable if changed, but they may be visible even if normal
Splenic	Along the splenic vein	From 3 to 5; 0.5–4 cm	Cranial abdomen, to the left (5), following the spleen course in the middle abdomen	The landmark is the splenic hilum; lymph nodes are aligned along the splenic vein. They are visible if changed

	TABLE 9.2			
	Parietal lymph nodes			
Lymph nodes	Anatomical site	Number and size (length)	Probe position	Ultrasound landmarks
Lumboaortic	Along the course of abdominal aorta and caudal vena cava, from diaphragm to the deep circumflex artery	Very small (<1 cm), from zero up to 17	Along the mid-line, starting from position 1 up to 7	Explore the region adjacent to the abdominal aorta and caudal vena cava, until the deep circumflex artery. Visible only if much changed, their finding is often associated to lymphoma
Renal	Close to the renal vessels	1 per side, sometimes absent; 1.5 cm	Middle abdomen, positions 3 and 10	Identify the aorta, the caudal vena cava and the confluence of renal arteries and renal veins, then explore surrounding mesenteric tissue. They are visible if changed
Medial iliac	Between the deep circumflex artery and the external iliac artery, laterally to the last part of the abdominal aorta and the caudal vena cava	Usually single, it may be double; 4–6 cm	Caudal abdomen, from position 1 move slightly to the right and the left of the mid-line. With the dog in right lateral recumbency, keep the probe close to the ventral edge of lumbar vertebral bodies. To evaluate the right portion of the aorta, changing the patient recumbency is better	Search for the emersion from the aorta of the deep circumflex artery and the external iliac artery, then explore the mesenteric tissue to the left and to the right of the aorta. If you have trouble, the transverse scan is very useful, as the vessel (anechoic lumen) is well differentiated from the lymph node (hypoechoic structure). They are almost always visible
Hypogastric	The angle formed by the sacral artery and internal iliac arteries.	From 1 to 3	More caudally to the previous position, towards the pelvis, over the aortic trifurcation	Iliac arteries are identified together with the sacral artery, which continues the aorta on the longitudinal plane. The tissue triangle between these vessels is explored. They are only visible if changed
Sacral	Close to the median sacral artery	Present in 50% of cases; <2 cm	More caudally to the previous position, towards the pelvis	The landmark is the sacral artery, they are difficult to see as much caudal (intrapelvic position)

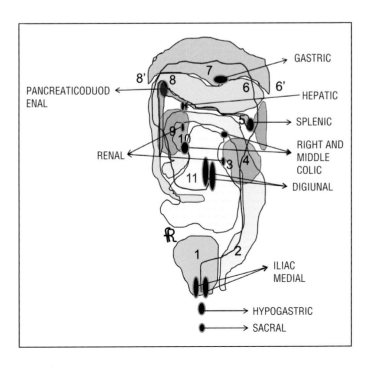

Figure 9.1 Localization of major abdominal lymph nodes.

ultrasonography. Table 9.3 groups superficial lymph nodes that can be visualized on ultrasonography.

VISIBILITY OF ABDOMINAL LYMPH NODES

In **dogs**, lymph nodes that are always easily visualized, even if normal, are jejunal lymph nodes (Fig. 9.1) and medial iliac lymph nodes (Fig. 9.2); so, a complete ultrasonographic examination must always include these structures. Right colic lymph nodes can be visualized in most dogs; however, this may also depend on repletion of large intestine and operator experience.

In particularly favourable conditions and suitable dogs, other lymph nodes (portal, splenic, middle colic, gastric) are sometimes visualized, even if normal, and these lymph nodes become easily visible when enlarged (Fig. 9.3, 9.4 and 9.5). The last group (caudal mesenteric, pancreaticoduodenal, aortic, renal, hypogastric and sacral lymph nodes) includes smaller and less easily retrievable lymph nodes, that become evident only if clearly enlarged.

In **cats**, normal lymph nodes are smaller and their visualization less common.

SIZE AND SHAPE OF ABDOMINAL LYMPH NODES

The length of abdominal lymph nodes is variable from about 1 cm to more than 6 cm, depending on their shape and location (see tables). On the contrary, the variability is reduced considering the thickness of normal lymph nodes, which is usually less than 1 centimetre. The normal form is elongated, with long-axis/short-axis ratio in clear favour of the former.

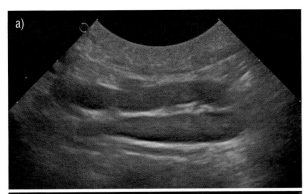
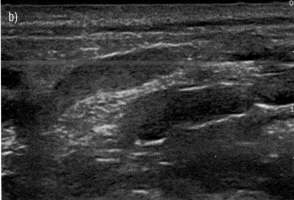

Figure 9.2   Normal jejunal lymph nodes; image obtained with a microconvex **(a)** and a linear **(b)** probe. Lymph nodes have elongated shapes and are echogenic and homogeneous on average.

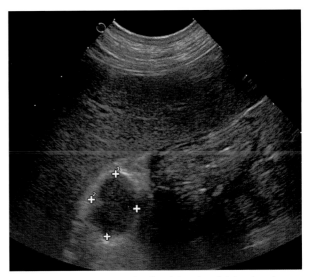

Figure 9.4   Reactive gastric lymph node in a dog; slightly enlarged, hypoechoic and homogeneous, surrounded by hyperechoic peritoneum.

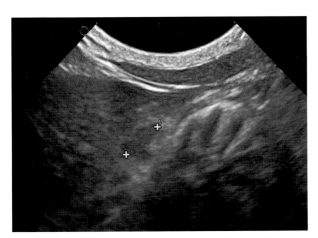

Figure 9.3   Normal gastric lymph node in a cat; small, normal in echogenicity and echostructure, surrounded by normal peritoneal fat.

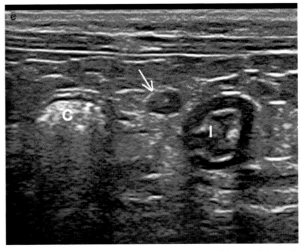

Figure 9.5   Normal right colic lymph node in a cat (white arrow); located close to the ileocolic junction, between the end portion of the ileum (I) and the ascending colon (C).

TABLE 9.3 Superficial lymph nodes				
Lymph nodes	Anatomical site	Number and size (length)	Probe position	Ultrasound landmarks
HEAD AND NECK REGION				
Mandibular	A bit ventrally to the angle of the mandible, at the confluence of the linguofacial vein in the external jugular vein	2 or 3 per side; about 1 cm	Superficial position, just ventrally to the angle of the mandible, on the left and the right	Follow the external jugular vein in the cranial direction until its termination. Another landmark is the mandibular salivary gland; lymph nodes are located just caudally to it
Medial retropharyngeal	Medially to the mandibular salivary gland, between this and the common carotid artery	1 per side; up to 5 cm in length	Start from the location identified for mandibular lymph nodes, then move slightly in the rostral direction	When you find the huge mandibular salivary gland, explore its medial region, laterally to the common carotid artery
Superficial cervical	Cranially to the scapulohumeral joint, laterally to ventral serratus and scalene muscles	1 per side; about 3 cm in length	Palpate the cranial edge of the scapulohumeral joint, then put the probe cranially to this	Explore the area cranially to the shoulder, between muscle bundles and fat
FORELIMB REGION				
Axillary	Axillary region, between the forelimb and thoracic wall	Usually 1 per side, sometimes 2; 2 cm	Place the probe in the axillary space	Axillary vessels are the landmark (axillary artery and vein), lymph nodes are in the fat surrounding these vessels
INGUINAL REGION				
Superficial inguinal	Caudal inguinal region; in adipose tissue located between the caudal abdominal wall and the medial surface of the tight. In females, lymph nodes are deeper than the mammary gland	1 or 2; 2 cm	Place the probe into the left or right inguinal region, over the abdominal wall, slightly medially to the tight, in males, slightly cranially to the scrotum	Identify the parenchyma of the last mammary gland; the lymph node is in the adipose tissue, deeper compared to the mammary gland
HINDLIMB REGION				
Superficial popliteal	The region caudal to the knee joint, in the fat between biceps femoris and semitendinosus muscles	Single; 2 cm	Place the probe in the caudal region of the knee	Search for any fat accumulation between biceps femoris and semitendinosus muscles

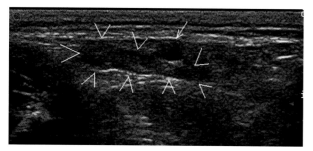

Figure 9.6 Normal mandibular lymph node (delimited by arrowheads). The arrow indicates the adjacent venous blood vessel (linguofacial vein).

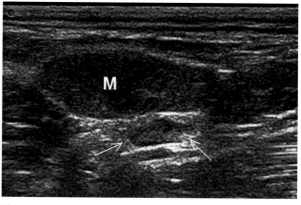

Figure 9.7 Normal medial retropharyngeal lymph node. The lymph node (arrows) is deeper and medially to the mandibular salivary gland (M).

TABLE 9.4
Ultrasonographic parameters useful to differentiate normal, inflammatory and neoplastic lymph nodes

Lymph nodes	Normal	Inflammatory	Neoplastic
Shape	elongated	elongated/oval	rounded
Long-axis/short-axis ratio	<0.55	<0.55	>0.55
Echogenicity	isoechoic	isoechoic/ slightly hypoechoic	hypoechoic
Echostructure	homogeneous	variable	heterogeneous/ variable
Hilar sign	present	often present	absent
Edges	variable	variable	clear
Blood flow distribution	hilar	hilar	Peripheral

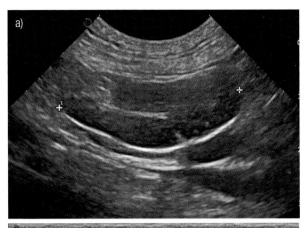

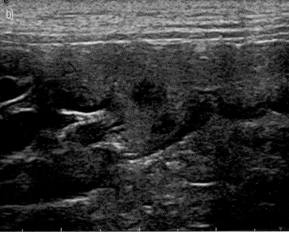

Figure 9.10 Reactive lymph nodes, slightly enlarged, long-axis/short axis ratio unchanged, slightly hypoechoic homogeneous **(a)** or hypoechoic heterogeneous with anechoic areas **(b)**.

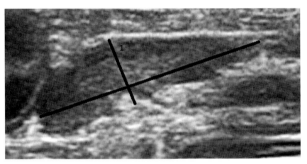

Figure 9.8 Long-axis/short-axis ratio in a normal lymph node, strongly in favour of the long axis (<0.55).

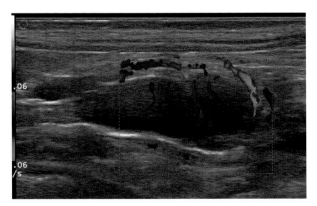

Figure 9.9 Normal Doppler flow of a lymph node; the normal hilar flow is visualized.

LYMPH NODES ULTRASONOGRAPHIC CHANGES

They can be found in primary or secondary, benign (e.g. inflammatory) or malignant (neoplastic) lymphadenopaties.

Differentiating a reactive lymph node from a neoplastic one is not always easy, especially when they are not much enlarged.

Table 9.4 shows some ultrasonographic parameters useful to differentiate normal, inflammatory and neoplastic lymph nodes.

Referring to Table 9.4, some important considerations are:

- The association between abnormal enlargement, significant changes in the long-axis/short axis ratio, rounded shape and decreased echogenicity of the lymph nodes parenchyma may prove significant **malignancy indexes**.
- The **hilar sign** is caused by hyperechoic adipose tissue in the lymph node medulla; its absence is attributed to changes in the normal echostructure during neoplastic phenomena; from an ultrasonographic point of view, the presence or absence of this sign is not significant to differentiate inflammatory and neoplastic lymph nodes.
- The **edges** evaluation is a highly variable parameter, often difficult to assess and therefore sometimes not very reliable.
- The parenchyma **heterogeneous** echostructure can be associated both to inflammatory and neoplastic forms (Fig. 9.12 and 9.13), and is caused by cystic or necrotic areas. The heterogeneity must not be considered indicative of malignancy, but is often associated to reactive forms, especially in cats.
- The **blood flow distribution**, which can be studied both with Colour Doppler or Contrast Enhanced Ultra-Sonography (CEUS), is most often hilar in inflammatory forms, and more often peripheral in neoplastic forms. Indeed, in malignant diseases we often have deviations of

one or more vessels with respect to the lymph node central axis; moreover, pericapsular or subcapsular vessels can arise from the capsule but without connection with longitudinal or central hilar vessels of the lymph node.

- Colour Doppler can also be important to differentiate a vessel from an anechoic/hypoechoic lymph node (for

example, medial iliac lymph nodes from the aorta and caudal vena cava); evaluating patients with tachypnea or particularly deep abdominal lymph nodes can be tricky and difficult.

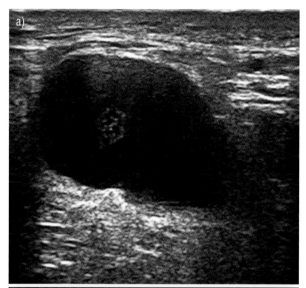

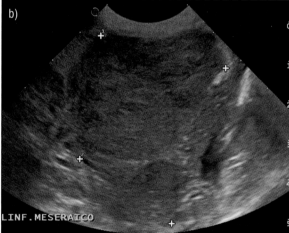

Figure 9.11   Neoplastic lymph nodes that are very enlarged and rounded (long-axis/short-axis ratio >0.55), hypoechoic, homogeneous **(a)**, or more heterogeneous **(b)**.

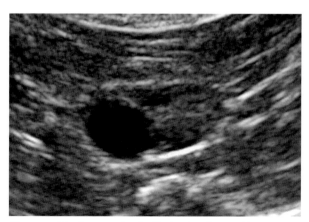

Figure 9.12   Heterogeneity of an iliac lymph node, caused by an anechoic cyst, which also warps the shape.

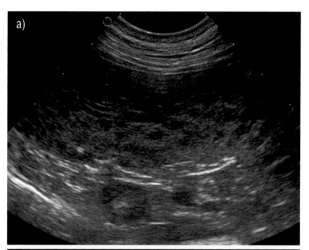

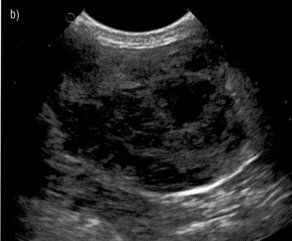

Figure 9.13   Heterogeneous neoplastic lymph nodes. **a)** Enlarged and heterogeneous splenic lymph node, due to lymphomatous infiltration in a dog. Note the typical hypoechoic and heterogeneous spleen appearance. **b)** Metastatic lymph node (prostatic carcinoma) with hypoechoic areas caused by haemorrhage and necrosis.

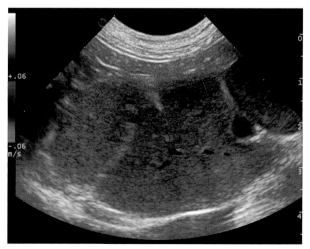

Figure 9.14   Lymphoma in a dog. Colour Doppler examination of a jejunal lymph node; changes in lymph node vascular architecture are visible.

The systematic ultrasonographic evaluation of the abdomen allows differentiation between a generalized lymphadenopathy and involvement of a single lymph node.

NEOPLASTIC FORMS

- In patients with lymphoma, a generalized lymphadenomegaly (less common, the involvement of a single lymph node) is often visible, often associated with extranodal changes as well; for example, cats with alimentary lymphoma may have single, or more often multiple, injuries in one or more intestinal loops, in the liver and/or the spleen, in addition to lymph node involvement (in particular, colic and mesenteric lymph nodes).
- Less often, the abdominal lymphadenopathy is associated with other types of multicentric neoplasms (e.g. malignant histiocytoma or mast cell tumour).
- A localized neoplasm requires the study of regional lymph nodes, both visceral and superficial. In mammary neoplasms that affect the caudal and/or inguinal breasts, or neoplasms/infections of the prostate or the bladder, it is very important to evaluate in particular the medial iliac lymph nodes, the hypogastric and sacral lymph nodes; less often lumbar aortic lymph nodes are affected. The lymphocentres themselves can also be involved in cutaneous and subcutaneous neoplasms of hindlimbs (e.g. mast cell tumours or sarcomas). In liver diseases portal lymph nodes are to be accurately assessed, while with spleen injuries the same applies to splenic lymph nodes.

INFLAMMATORY FORMS

Inflammatory conditions often cause reactive lymphadenopathy of satellite regional lymph nodes; for example, in inflammatory bowel diseases jejunal lymph nodes are involved.

However, some infectious diseases (for example, leishmaniasis in dogs or PIF in cats) are associated with generalized lymphadenopathy.

For a definitive diagnosis of benign or malignant lymphadenopathy it is still essential to perform an ultrasound-guided cytological and/or histological examination of lymph nodes, a simple method that allows one to obtain reliable results with limited procedural risks.

RECOMMENDED READING

Pugh CR. Ultrasonographic examination of abdominal lymph nodes in the dog. Vet Radiol Ultrasound 1994. 35: 110–115.

Schreurs E, Vermote K, Barberet V, et al. Ultrasonographic anatomy of abdominal lymph nodes in the normal cat. Vet Radiol Ultrasound 2008, 49(1): 68–72.

Nyman HT, Kristensen AT, Flagstad A, et al. A review of the sonographic assessment of tumor metastases in liver and superficial lymph nodes. Vet Radiol Ultrasound 2004, 45: 438–448.

Agthe P, Caine AR, Posch B. Ultrasonographic appearance of jejunal lymph nodes in dogs without clinical signs of gastrointestinal disease. Vet Rad Ultrasound 2009, 50: 195–200.

Llabres-Diaz FJ. Ultrasonography of the medial iliac lymph nodes in the dog. Vet Radiol Ultrasound 2004. 45: 156–165.

Nyman HT, Kristensen AT, Skovgaard IM, et al. Characterization of normal and abnormal canine superficial lymph nodes using gray-scale bmode, color flow mapping, power, and spectral doppler ultrasonography: a multivariate study. Vet Radiol Ultrasound 2005, 46: 404–410.

De Swarte M, Alexander K, Rannou B, et al. Comparison of sonographic features of benign and neoplastic deep lymph nodes in dogs. Vet Radiol Ultrasound 2011.

Kinns J, Mai W. Association between malignancy and sonographic heterogeneity in canine and feline abdominal lymph nodes. Vet Radiol Ultrasound 2007. 48: 565–569.

Prieto S, Gomez-Ochoa P, De Blas I, et al. Pathologic correlation of resistive and pulsatility indices in canine abdominal lymph nodes. Vet Radiol Ultrasound 2009. (50): 525–529.

Gelb HR, Freeman LJ, Rohleder JJ, et al. Feasibility of contrast-enhanced ultrasound-guided biopsy of sentinel lymph nodes in dogs. Vet Radiol Ultrasound 2010. 51: 628–633.

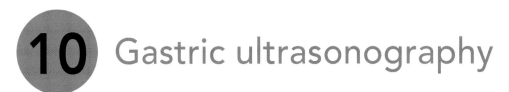

10 Gastric ultrasonography

Edoardo Auriemma

SCAN TECHNIQUE (Fig. 10.1–2)

Animal preparation	• 12 hours on an empty stomach, at least. • Wide hair-clipping, including intercostal spaces. • Dorsal recumbency, right lateral (best visualization of pyloric antrum) and/or left lateral (best visualization of fundus), quadrupedal posture (best visualization of pylorus and body). Changing animal recumbencies helps in exploring different stomach areas, as the gas moves away from the area of interest, providing a better acoustic window.
Probes	• Microconvex, 5 MHz mean frequency (3–8 MHz). • Linear, high-frequency (7.5–12 MHz), for small breed animals and organ superficial portions.

(Continued →)

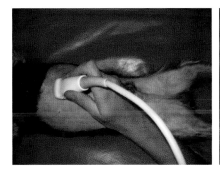

Figure 10.1a Position 7; just caudally to the liver visceral edge where the body of the stomach is located.

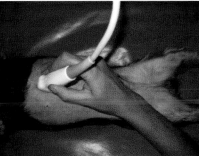

Figure 10.1b Position 7; from the transverse scan, the probe is rotated counter-clockwise by 90 degrees. The gastric axis is different in dogs and cats.

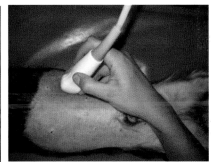

Figure 10.1c Position 6, oblique scan directed on the left. This position allows for evaluation of the gastric fundus.

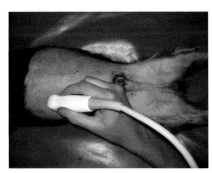

Figure 10.1d Position 8, oblique scan directed on the right. This position allows for evaluation of the pyloric antrum. A right intercostal scan is sometimes preferable to evaluate the passage between pylorus and duodenum.

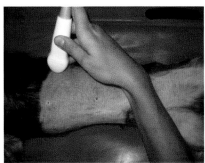

Figure 10.1e Position 6; left intercostal scan. This position allows for evaluation of the gastric fundus, especially in large breed dogs.

SCAN TECHNIQUE (Continued)

Scans and respective probe position	

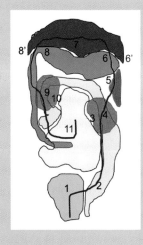	• Transverse scan (position 7): The probe on the median line, in contact with the xyphoid process of the sternum, the beam oriented transversely with mild cranial tilt to identify the liver (Fig. 10.1a).
	
	    Reducing the cranial rocking and putting the probe a bit more perpendicular, the liver visceral edge is identified; the stomach lies just caudally to this edge.
	• DOG: The stomach is in the centre of the cranial abdomen and one of its axes is nearly perpendicular to the spine.
	• CAT: The stomach is on the left of the cranial abdomen and one of its axes is perpendicular to the spine.
	• Longitudinal scan (position 7): with the probe in contact with the xyphoid process of the sternum and the beam directed longitudinally, start from a middle position then move right and left (Fig. 10.1b).
	• Oblique scans (positions 6 and 8): move the probe from position 7 to position 6 (Fig. 10.1c) and finally to position 8 (Fig. 10.1d), gliding along the costal arch and tilting the probe left and right.
	• Intercostal scans (positions 6' and 8'): the probe is over the last two intercostal spaces; it is useful to visualize the pyloric region (8') to the right, and the fundic area (6') to the left (Fig. 10.1e).
	• Indicated mainly in deep-chest dogs.
	• The transition between pylorus and proximal duodenum is not always easy to visualize, especially in dogs (Fig. 10.2).
	
	    The best approach is a longitudinal scan of the right cranial abdomen: with the probe along the abdominal wall, the proximal duodenum is identified and followed cranially until a dorsal curvature which corresponds to the pyloric region.

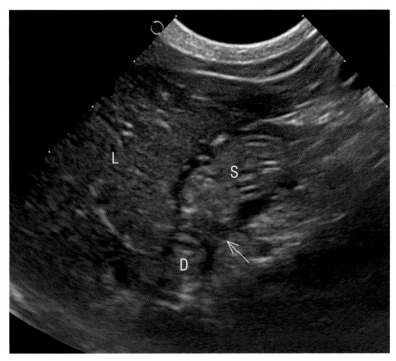

Figure 10.2 Transition between pylorus and duodenum. In dogs, due to the almost perpendicular tilt between pylorus and proximal duodenum, images are often ill-defined.

ULTRASONOGRAPHIC ANATOMY (Fig. 10.3–5)

Location	Middle cranial abdomen, right and left, just caudally to the liver.
Morphology (Fig. 10.3)	**Hollow organ, 3 separate regions:** • **Fundus**: identifiable by its localization in the left abdomen and typical gastric folds (Fig. 10.3). • Gastric folds of the fundic region are the most developed; however, they are more or less visible depending on distension degree and type of gastric contents. On an empty stomach they tend to collapse and become more noticeable (especially in cats); if the stomach is distended, they are not visible on ultrasonography. • Sometimes the cardia and distal esophagus are visible next to the diaphragm, slightly displaced to the left. The visibility depends on patient conformation, degree of gastric repletion and stomach contents. • **Body**: it is in a central abdominal position, gastric folds are less developed, the transition between fundus and body is ill-defined. • **Pyloric antrum/pylorus**: it is in the right abdomen in dogs, in the central abdomen in cats; folds are underdeveloped. • The transverse diameter is very reduced, the wall is thicker, especially the muscular coat component. In the transition between duodenum and pylorus, especially in cats, the thickness and echogenicity of the submucosa are increased, as well as the thickness of the muscular coat (Fig. 11.8, Chapter 11).
Relationships with adjacent organs evaluable on ultrasonography	• **Cranially**: liver. • **Caudally to the left**: spleen, left lobe of the pancreas. • **Caudally to the right**: duodenum, right lobe of the pancreas. • **Caudally to the centre**: body of the pancreas, transverse colon.

Size	• Highly variable, depending on gastric distension degree.
	• Mean parietal thickness: it varies according to point of measurement (intra-fold or inter-folds), gastric distension and subject size. By convention, the gastric wall is measured between folds and its mean size reported in the literature is:
	  – 3–5 mm (dog)
	  – 2–2.2 mm (cat).

Echogenicity	• Gastric wall: regular, well-defined, layered.
	• There are five identifiable layers that proceed from the esophagus to the rectum and are more easy to visualize in the small intestine (Fig. 11.2, Chapter 11).
	From the outside towards the lumen they are:
	  – Hyperechoic line: serous coat
	  – Hypoechoic layer: muscular coat
	  – Hyperechoic line: submucosa
	  – Hypoechoic layer: mucous coat
	  – Hyperechoic line: mucous coat–gastric lumen interface.
	• Content: it varies depending on the content
	  – Mucous pattern: thin hyperechoic line (Fig. 10.3)
	  – Fluid pattern (anechoic, hypoechoic) (Fig. 10.4)
	  – Gaseous pattern: hyperechoic with reverberation artefact (Fig. 10.5)
	  – Mixed pattern: variable echogenicity, reverberation artefacts and posterior shadowing (fluid, gas, ingesta).

Echostructure	• Homogeneous in all parietal layers.
Peristalsis	• 4–6 peristaltic movements per minute.
Tributary lymph nodes	• Gastric. • Hepatic. • Splenic.

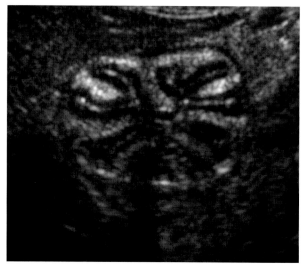

Figure 10.3 Normal gastric parietal stratigraphy of the fundic region in a cat on an empty stomach.

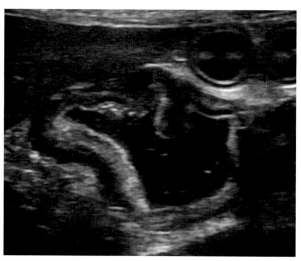

Figure 10.4 Fluid gastric contents: if smallest, it allows for a better visualization of gastric stratigraphy and folds.

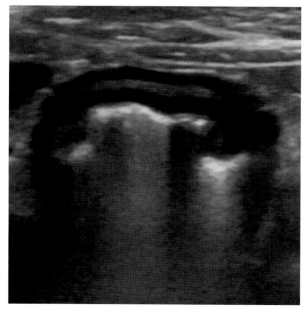

Figure 10.5 Gaseous gastric contents associated with reverberation artefact.

ULTRASONOGRAPHIC CHANGES: GASTRIC DISEASES

Gastric diseases of ultrasonographic interest can be classified into three groups:

- Inflammatory diseases
- Neoplastic diseases
- Obstructive diseases.

The ultrasonographic examination must be systematic, paying particular attention to: thickness, stratigraphy, wall symmetry, content, motility, appearance of peritoneum and surrounding fat, regional lymph nodes.

INFLAMMATORY DISEASES
DIFFUSE: gastritis.
FOCAL: gastric ulcer, gastric abscesses.

GASTRITIS (Fig. 10.6–7)
The patient must be evaluated on an empty stomach and without any gastric distension.

Different ultrasonographic scans are selected and extra care is needed to differentiate the normal parietal plication with a pathological thickening. In doubtful cases, administering water to the patient before the stomach assessment can be useful to obtain an adequate parietal distension which ensures more accurate measurements. Unfortunately, especially in dogs and even under best conditions, it is not always possible to evaluate the entire gastric wall.

Ultrasonographic findings in acute gastritis (Fig. 10.6):

- The stomach may appear normal on ultrasonography; as an alternative, the wall can be only slightly thickened and the stratigraphy preserved
- Parietal changes are more marked if associated with wall **oedema**; in these cases, the thickening is bigger and can be associated with changes in the parietal stratigraphy, thin hypoechoic edge just beneath the lumen–mucous coat interface, and thickening of the submucosa, less echoic than the norm (Fig. 10.7)
- In many cases, the inflammation-associated atony reduces the peristalsis causing the accumulation of material in the gastric lumen (often fluid)
- Possible gastric ulcers (see below).

In case of **chronic** gastritis, ultrasonographic findings include:

- Moderate and diffuse parietal thickening
- Possible change in parietal echogenicity, but preserved stratigraphy
- In case of uraemic gastropathy, mineralization of the mucous coat which appears as a hyperechoic line at the mucous coat-gastric lumen interface (Fig. 10.8)
- Occasionally, fluid gastric contents
- Decreased gastric motility.

GASTRIC ULCER (Fig. 10.9–10)
Gastric ulcers are complications of inflammatory or neoplastic diseases. The localization of injury, often focal, requires a careful evaluation of the gastric wall, and the absence of any ultrasonographic finding does not exclude a possible injury.

In doubtful cases it is recommended to complete the evaluation of patients with the endoscopic examination and possibly the gastric biopsy.

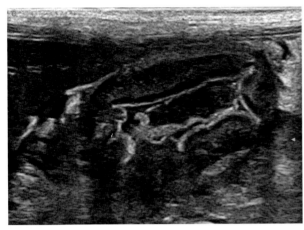

Figure 10.6 Very severe thickening of the gastric wall in a dog with acute gastritis (parvovirosis). The lumen contains some fluid and a hyperechoic linear structure reportable to partial mucosal avulsion.

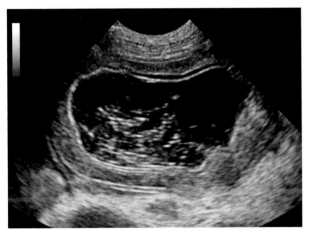

Figure 10.7 Parietal oedema, recognizable as a thin hypoechoic band, interfaced to a thicker submucosa, less echoic than normal.

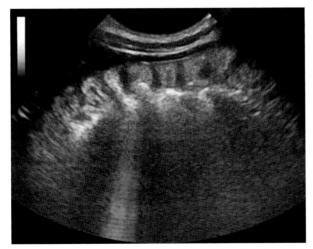

Figure 10.8 Hyperechogenicity of the lumen-gastric wall interface in case of chronic uremic gastritis.

ULTRASONOGRAPHIC FINDINGS
- Hypoechoic focal parietal thickening with irregularity of the mucosal edge (ulcer crater) (Fig. 10.9)
- Loss of stratigraphy (focal) (Fig. 10.10)

- Intramural gas that appears as a hyperechoic area associated with typical reverberation artefacts
- Reduced peristalsis with fluid gastric contents
- Hyperechogenicity of surrounding mesentery (Fig. 10.9)
- In case of gastric perforation, a small layer of effusion next to the injury, and/or pneumoperitoneum.

GASTRIC ABSCESSES (Fig. 10.11)
- Often associated with penetrating foreign bodies
- Intra-extramural neoformations with dominant corpuscular fluid contents (Fig. 10.11)
- Usually associated with gastric parietal changes and peritonitis
- Differential diagnosis: neoplasm.

NEOPLASTIC DISEASES
DIFFUSE – Statistically, the most common ones are: lymphoma (especially in cats), mast cell tumour (systemic form). FOCAL – Statistically, the most common ones are: adenocarcinoma

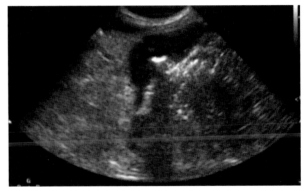

Figure 10.9 Typical appearance of a gastric ulcer: focal hypoechoic parietal thickening associated with loss of stratigraphy. At the centre there is a depression (crater) with trapped gas (hyperechoic interface). Note the mesentery hyperechogenicity associated to the gastric wall affected by the ulcer.

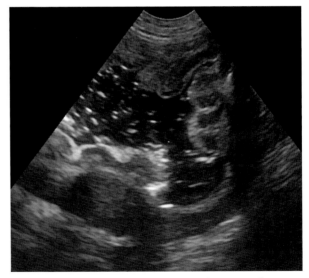

Figure 10.10 Wide gastric ulcer with a crater that contains plenty of gas (two hyperechoic lines to the left of the crater); nevertheless, echoic material covers the crater floor (probably necrotic material). Note that, around the ulcer, the gastric wall is considerably thickened, hypoechoic and lacking normal stratigraphy.

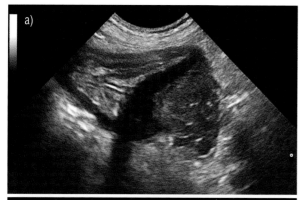

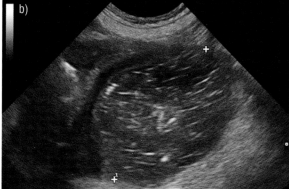

Figure 10.11 Intraparietal a) and extraluminal b) gastric abscess with well-defined wall and echoic corpuscular content. Note the hyperechogenicity of surrounding peritoneum.

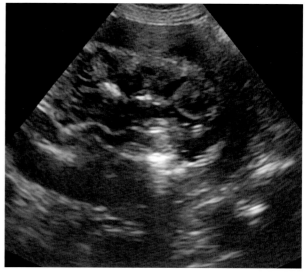

Figure 10.12 Severe parietal thickening of the antrum region with altered stratigraphy (pseudostratigraphy). There is some intraparietal gas due to an ulcer. Final diagnosis: gastric carcinoma.

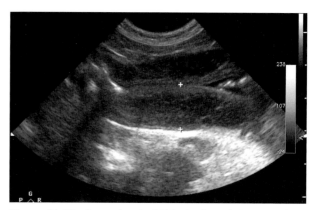

Figure 10.13 Concentric parietal thickening, hypoechoic, associated with loss of stratigraphy: gastric lymphoma.

(especially in dogs), lymphoma (especially in cats), leiomyoma/leiomyosarcoma.

Other focal lesions are gastric polyps; they are benign injuries but must be differentiated from malignant neoplasms. The differentiation between these neoplasms cannot rely on ultrasonography only, but must be confirmed by cytology/histology.

ADENOCARCINOMAS/CARCINOMAS (Fig. 10.12)
- As a general rule, the carcinoma tends to be more localized and smaller (as symptoms are more precocious) compared to lymphoma; moreover, it tends to extend intraluminally causing more often an occlusion
- Sometimes, especially in carcinomas, there is a particular change in the normal stratigraphy of the gastric wall, the so-called 'pseudolayering'. In pseudolayering, the changed wall shows alternating hypoechoic and hyperechoic layers that do not fulfil the normal ultrasonographic anatomy (Fig. 10.12)
- Preferential location: lesser curvature and antrum
- Often, regional lymph nodes (gastric, hepatic and splenic) are hypoechoic, rounded, possibly enlarged and surrounded by hyperechoic mesentery
- Possible injuries in other abdominal organs.

LYMPHOMA (Fig. 10.13)
- Focal, multifocal, or diffuse (circumferential) parietal thickening
- Loss of normal parietal stratigraphy
- Often, hypoechoic or anechoic wall
- Usually, no intraluminal spread

- Regional adenopathy a bit less common compared to the carcinoma, but often present
- Possible injuries in other abdominal organs.

LEIOMYOMAS/LEIOMYOSARCOMAS
- Neoplasms originating from the muscular coat (leiomyoma/leiomyosarcoma) tend to expand eccentrically, i.e. outwardly, maintaining the gastric lumen pervious for long; this is why patients are long-lasting asymptomatic and these masses are diagnosed when they have reached considerable size
- If they are at pylorus level, can cause obstruction
- Focal asymmetrical parietal thickening
- Preferential localization: the cardia
- Parietal echogenicity often decreased, with loss of normal parietal stratigraphy
- More uncommon, regional lymph nodes and other abdominal organs are involved.

GASTRIC POLYPS (Fig. 10.14)
In asymptomatic patients they are often accidental findings. Polyps are benign adenomatous mucosal neoformations, commonly in the antral location, projecting in the gastric lumen.

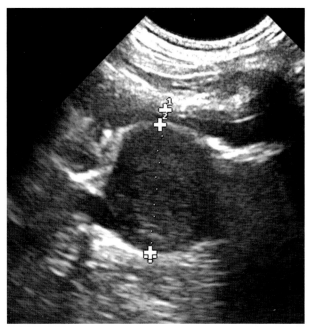

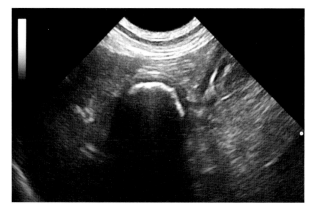

Figure 10.15 Hyperechoic curved interface followed by clean posterior shadowing. This is the typical finding of a gastric foreign body.

Figure 10.14 Gastric polyp; echoic, well-defined and benign injury. The final diagnosis is always histological. They must be differentiated from gastric neoplasms.

- Hyperechoic parietal or mixed echogenicity injuries (Fig. 10.14)
- Gastric stratigraphy is usually preserved (barring very massive injuries or those associated to severe parietal oedema)
- Mainly pyloric localization
- Possible partial gastric obstruction
- Usually, no regional lymphadenopathy
- Differential diagnosis: gastric neoplasm; cytological/ histological examination recommended.

OBSTRUCTIVE DISEASES (Fig. 10.15)

Gastric occlusion and subocclusion may be secondary to mechanical causes (foreign bodies, neoplasms, polyps, gastroduodenal intussusception, congenital or acquired pyloric hypertrophy) or functional causes (pylorospasm or paralytic ileus). To investigate a patient with gastric obstruction and try to find the cause, changing the patient recumbency during the examination is useful; this way, fluid and gas move helping to highlight the obstructive injury. In case of suspected pyloric obstruction, the patient is best positioned in right lateral recumbency, and studied with the probe in positions 8 and 8'.

So, the fluid goes down in the stomach declivous portion (pyloric region) allowing for a better injury visualization.

Sometimes, keeping the patient over a cardiology examination table and using its declivous openings can help to reach position 8'.

ULTRASONOGRAPHIC FINDINGS

- Distended stomach with mixed fluid–gas content
- Absent to ineffective motility, with gastric material that is mixed but does not move in the aboral direction
- Ultrasound reflective foreign bodies (metal, wood, plastic, bones, stones) appear as differently shaped and sized interfaces (hyperechoic bands) with clean posterior shadowing (different from that emitted by gas) (Fig. 10.15)
- Some foreign bodies (fabric, trichobezoars, phytobezoars) can be often confused with food material due to their composition, shape, ability to entrap the air. In this case, fasting the animal (24–48 h) is recommended before repeating the ultrasonographic examination
- Linear foreign bodies can pass through the stomach and cause abnormal plication
- In doubtful cases, an abdominal radiographic study is recommended as complementary examination.

RECOMMENDED READING

Martha Moon Larson, David S. Biller: Ultrasound of the gastrointestinal tract. Vet Clin Small Anim 2009, 39: 747–759.

Hoffman KL: Sonographic signs of gastroduodenale linear foreign body in 3 dogs. Vet Radiol Ultrasound. 2003, 44: 466–469.

Lamb CR, Grierson J. Ultrasonographic appearance of primary gastric neoplasia in 21 dogs. J Small Anim Pract. 1999, 40(5): 211–215.

Penninck D, Matz M, Tidwell A 1997. Ultrasonography of gastric ulceration in the dog.

Grooters AM, Miyabayashi T, Biller Ds, Merryma J: Sonographic appearance of uremic gastropathy in four dogs. Veterinary Radiology & Ultrasound. 1994, 35(1): 35–40.

11 Bowel ultrasonography

Giliola Spattini

SCAN TECHNIQUE (Fig. 11.1)

Animal preparation	• 12–24 hours on an empty stomach, at least. • Wide hair-clipping, including intercostal spaces. • Dorsal recumbency, right and left lateral recumbency or quadrupedal posture.
Probes	• Microconvex, 7.5 MHz mean frequency. • Linear, high-frequency (10–14 MHz) for small breed animals and more superficial intestinal loops.
Scans and respective probe position 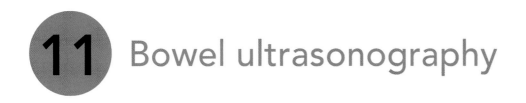	**Proximal duodenum:** • **Transverse scan** (position 8'): patient preferably in left lateral recumbency. The probe is over the 9th (±1) intercostal space, transversely oriented, ventrally to the visceral edge of the liver (Fig. 11.1a). A small intestine loop is visible between the liver surface and the abdominal wall of the right flank, with very prominent mucous coat (especially in dogs), which cranially continues in the pylorus. • **Longitudinal scan** (position 8): starting from the transverse scan, the probe is rotated by 90 degrees (Fig. 11.1b). In patients with a chest that is not very deep, the subcostal scan can be used rather than the intercostal one (Fig. 11.1c). To get good quality images staying perpendicular to the organ under examination is needed, with the probe kept parallel to the ultrasonographic table plane. A very light pressure on the probe is needed. • **Distal duodenum, jejunum, proximal ileum** (starting from position 11, explore the middle and caudal abdomen): intestinal loops are freely scattered in the abdominal cavity; there are no precise ultrasound landmarks. To evaluate all the enteric tract 'Greek fret' scans are used throughout the middle and caudal abdomen (Fig. 11.1d). Loops must be studied in the longitudinal and transverse scan. • **Ileocecocolic junction:** (caudomedially to position 9) the position varies but is generally located in the right hemiabdomen over the fourth lumbar vertebra (Fig. 11.1e). The medial and ventral region of the right kidney is explored to identify a colon loop. To find the junction, follow this loop a bit cranially or caudally with transverse scans, then study it with a longitudinal scan. It is very important to avoid excessive pressures on the abdominal wall, or the colon will move away. • **Colon:** the probe is moved along the organ course, from the ileocecocolic junction in the cranial direction, then to the left, and lastly caudally up to the pelvic canal (Fig. 11.1f). In the caudal abdomen it has a close anatomical relationship with the bladder (position 2). Transverse and longitudinal scans are performed; due to artefacts created by food content, most diagnostic images are obtained with transverse scans.

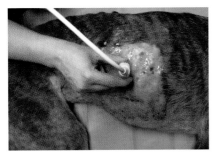

Figure 11.1a Patient in left lateral recumbency; the right flank is dorsal. The probe is over the central portion of the ninth intercostal space, with perpendicular tilting to the patient surface and transversely oriented beam.

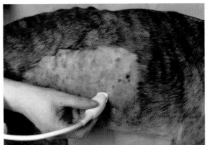

Figure 11.1b From position in Fig. 11.1a, the probe is rotated about 90 degrees and aligned with the duodenum longitudinal axis.

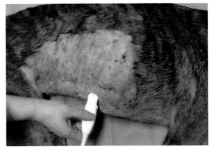

Figure 11.1c Subcostal scan. To get good quality images the probe must be perpendicular to the organ to be examined. The probe is parallel to the ultrasonographic table plane.

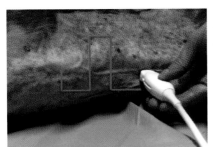

Figure 11.1d All abdomen quadrants are scanned systematically, drawing a 'Greek fret'. Both recumbencies are used, without missing any abdominal area.

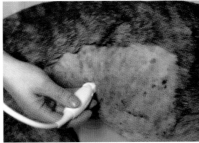

Figure 11.1e The probe is over the right hemiabdomen at the fourth lumbar vertebra level. Starting from a longitudinal scan of the right kidney, the probe is then moved medially and ventrally.

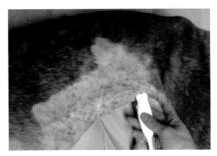

Figure 11.1f The probe is in the central portion of the caudal abdomen, over the linea alba. The probe is caudally translated until colon and bladder are identified.

ULTRASONOGRAPHIC ANATOMY (Fig. 11.2–10)

Location	• Proximal duodenum: right flank, cranial abdomen. • Distal duodenum, jejunum, proximal ileum: all middle and caudal abdomen. • Ileocecocolic junction: right hemiabdomen, on about the fourth lumbar vertebra. • Colon. ***Ascending:*** it originates from the ileocecocolic junction and moves cranially in the right hemiabdomen up to delimit the caudal edge of the pancreatic body. ***Transverse:*** it moves from the right hemiabdomen to the left one, then it goes very close to the stomach, caudal and parallel to it. ***Descending:*** in the left hemiabdomen it is located ventrally and medially to the spleen and the left kidney. It goes toward the pelvic canal remaining dorsal to the bladder.
Morphology	• **Parietal stratigraphy:** the whole gastrointestinal tract, from the esophagus to the colon, has a typical standard stratigraphy; the duodenum is the loop where the stratigraphy is best defined (Fig. 11.2). • **Proximal duodenum, Peyer's patches:** sometimes visible, but only in dogs, they appear as depressions in the antimesenteric edge of the proximal duodenum (Fig. 11.3). • **Caudal duodenum, jejunum and ileum:** they are difficult to differentiate: the duodenum has a slightly greater mucosal thickness; the ileum has a submucosa and a more prominent muscular coat compared to duodenum and jejunum. Differences are not always marked or significant. • **Ileocecocolic junction:** characteristic appearance (Fig. 11.4, 11.5) of an 'old-wagon wheel', especially in cats (submucosa and muscular coat are more prominent). If identifiable, the cecum course is more irregular and corrugated (it resembles a sausage) and short in length (Fig. 11.6). • **Colon:** it features a thin wall, large lumen and particular content: fecal material mixed with air, which creates characteristic artefacts (Fig. 11.7).

(Continued →)

ULTRASONOGRAPHIC ANATOMY (continued)

Relationships with adjacent organs evaluable on ultrasonography	• **Proximal duodenum:** cranially, it extends the pyloric canal (Fig. 11.8) and runs close to the pancreas body. In the intermediate portion it is in close relationship with the pancreas right lobe until about the cranial edge of the right kidney. In the same region it has a relationship with the ascending and transverse colon. A few centimetres after the beginning, the **major duodenal papilla** makes the common outlet for the bile duct and the pancreatic duct (Fig. 11.9). A few centimetres more caudally the **minor duodenal papilla** (Fig. 11.10) is visualized; it is the outlet of the accessory pancreatic duct (the most important and often the only duct in dogs, absent in most cats). • **Distal duodenum, jejunum, proximal ileum, ileocecocolic junction and colon:** these intestinal tracts have relationships with several adjacent organs as they do not have a fixed place but move freely in the abdomen.
Size	• The intestinal wall thickness changes according to the examined tract, the species and the age (see Table 11.1).
Edges	• Well-defined, clear and regular along the entire apparatus.
Echogenicity	• **Lumen–mucous coat interface:** depending on the lumen content, different ultrasonographic patterns are identified. • **Mucous coat:** hypoechoic or anechoic in all the enteric tract, with regular, well-defined, and smooth surface (Fig. 11.2). In a patient that has recently eaten, hyperechoic foci within the mucous coat (considered fat micelles under absorption) may be normal, while they must be absent in patients on an empty stomach. • **Submucosa:** uniformly thin, hyperechoic, well-defined compared to mucous coat and muscular coat (Fig. 11.2). The submucosa is usually more prominent in the ileum compared to jejunum and duodenum, especially in cats. • Muscular coat: hypoechoic, thinner than mucous coat. Uniform, well-defined, symmetrical (Fig. 11.2). Most prominent in ileum, especially in cats. • **Serous coat:** uniformly thin, hyperechoic, well-defined compared to muscular coat (Fig. 11.2). It marks the intestine from abdominal tissues.
Echostructure	• Homogeneous in all parietal layers.
Peristalsis	Small intestine: 3–5 peristaltic waves per minute on average. • Colon: generally, no primary peristaltic waves are identified as they are active only during defecation. • Peristaltic acts are identified by holding down the probe and observing propulsive movement of ingesta in the examined tract. This movement must be symmetrical, synchronous, effective.
Vessels	• **Cranial mesenteric artery and celiac artery**. The origin of these arteries from the aorta is a major landmark to identify adrenal glands and cranial mesenteric lymph nodes. These parallel vessels are visualized when they emerge from the aorta, just cranially to the origin of renal arteries. They are very close to each other and must be identified on the same scan plane. They supply blood to the cranial region of the colon, small intestine and stomach, as well as other abdominal viscera. • **Caudal mesenteric artery:** single, identifiable by Colour Doppler only, it originates from the ventral surface of the aorta, just cranially to the onset of two deep circumflex arteries, just ventrally to the intervertebral disc L5–6. It supplies with blood the caudal portion of the colon. • **Caudal mesenteric vein:** small sized, it drains most of the caudal surface of the large intestine and reaches the cranial mesenteric vein. • **Cranial mesenteric vein:** it drains most of the small intestine and the proximal surface of the large intestine. • The joining of the caudal mesenteric vein and the cranial mesenteric vein makes the portal vein that goes cranially towards the porta hepatis.
Tributary lymph nodes	• The main regional lymphocentres that are almost always identifiable even in healthy patients are the cranial mesenteric (or jejunal) lymph nodes and the right colic lymph nodes. Caudal mesenteric lymph nodes are identifiable if pathological.

TABLE 11.1
Wall thickness of the GI tract according to Penninck (2008) and Stander (2010)

Wall thickness in mm	Dog	Puppy	Cat
STOMACH	2–5 *	2.7 +/- 0.4 (2.2–3.7)	1.7–3.6
DUODENUM	3–6°	3.8 +/- 0.5 (3.2–4.8)	2.0–2.5
DUODENUM MUCOUS COAT		2.7 +/- 0.5 (2.0–3.8)	
JEJUNUM	2–5°	2.5 +/- 0.5 (1.2–3.4)	2.0–2.5
JEJUNUM MUCOUS COAT		1.5 +/- 0.4 (0.6–2.5)	
ILEUM	2–4		2.5–3.2
COLON	2–3	1.3 +/- 0.3 (0.7–2.0)	1.4–2.5

* = measurements taken between gastric folds; wide variations according to the gastric filling.
° = There is a correlation with the body weight.

TABLE 11.2
Mean percentages of intestinal coats in cats according to Winter (Abstract IVRA 2009)

	Stomach %	Duodenum %	Jejunum %	Ileum %
MUCOUS COAT	32	49	43	37
SUBMUCOSA	24	19	16	22
MUSCULAR COAT	24	17	22	25
SEROUS COAT	18	16	17	17

INTESTINE SYSTEMATIC EVALUATION

The intestine must be systematically evaluated for both parietal morphology and peristalsis. Parietal changes may be diffuse or localized, and must be typed on the basis of:

- Injury position
- Changes in parietal stratigraphy
- Injury symmetry
- Functional effect (reduction in parietal elasticity, paralytic or mechanical ileus, occlusion or subocclusion)

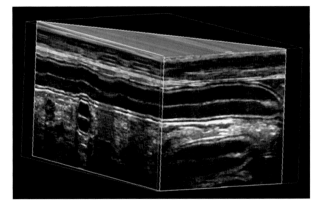

Figure 11.2 Three-dimensional reconstruction of a small intestine loop. Starting from inside to outside, the stratigraphy includes: hyperechoic lumen–mucous coat interface, anechoic mucous coat, thin and hyperechoic submucosa, hypoechoic muscular coat, and hyperechoic serous coat that marks off intestines from surrounding organs and tissues. The stratigraphy is well-defined and evident both in the longitudinal scan and the transverse scan.

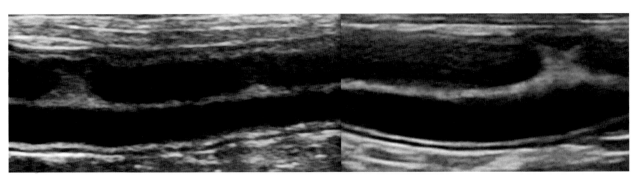

Figure 11.3 Peyer's patches in the duodenum of a dog.

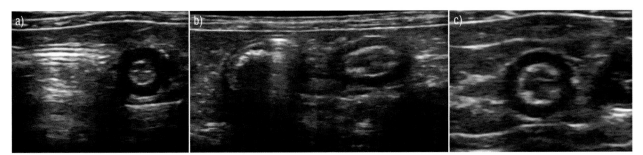

Figure 11.4 **a)** Transverse scan of the ileocecocolic junction of a cat, just before the ileum engages the ileocecocolic valve. At the ileocecocolic valve, the muscular coat appears thickened. **b)** Image just caudal to the previous one; the ileum is close to the colon. **c)** Image just cranial compared to the previous one; typical aspect of the cat ileum with very marked submucosa and muscular coat.

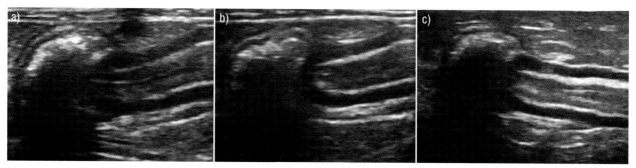

Figure 11.5 **a)** Longitudinal scan of the patient ileocecocolic valve of Fig. 11.4. **b)** Longitudinal scan corresponding to Fig. 11.8b. **c)** Longitudinal scan corresponding to Fig. 11.4c.

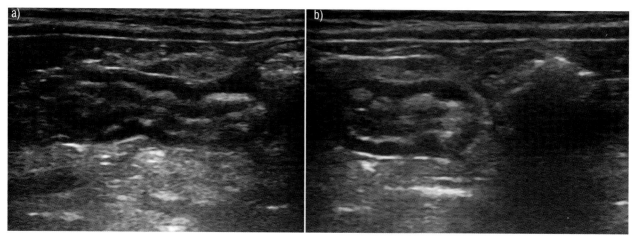

Figure 11.6 Just caudally and ventrally to the ileocolic valve, the cecocolic junction is found. When visible, cecum stratigraphy is similar to the ileum but corrugated. **a)** Longitudinal scan of a cat cecum, **b)** Transverse scan.

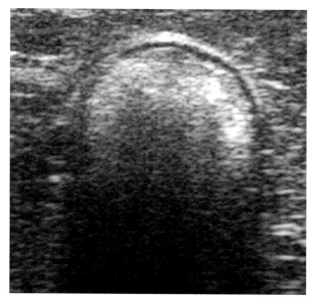

◄ **Figure 11.7** Transverse scan of the colon. Note that the fecal content, due to its gas content, creates a dirty acoustic shadow that hides the more distal wall.

Figure 11.8 **a)** Position 8. Just cranially and to the right of the pylorus, the duodenum originates. **b)** Image immediately caudal to the previous one; the hypoechoic portion separating the duodenum from the stomach is the prominent muscular coat of the pylorus. **c)** Image immediately caudal and to the left of the previous one, stomach-pylorus transition. Note the thickening of the muscular coat within the stomach-pylorus transition.
▼

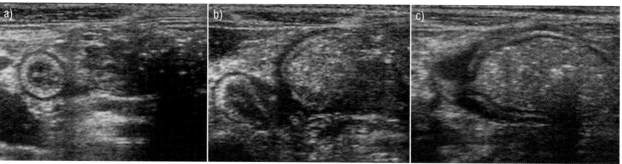

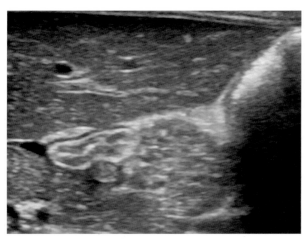

Figure 11.9 Major duodenal papilla in a cat. Note that it is rounded, well-defined and deviates from the duodenal wall. The pancreas is contiguous to this structure. Other identifiable organs are the liver and the colon. There is a clear small anechoic collection between duodenum and hepatic lobes.

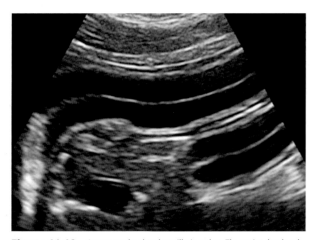

Figure 11.10 Accessory duodenal papilla in a dog. The major duodenal papilla is more cranial, and not identifiable in this image.

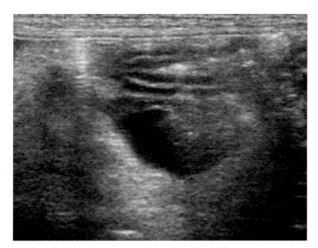

Figure 11.11 A patient with intestinal perforation. The image shows free air, characterized by a comet tail artefact. An anechoic collection looks in contact with an intestinal loop and surrounded by hyperechoic mesentery, with distal echoes dispersion.

- Peritoneal involvement
- Involvement of regional lymph nodes.

Gastric diseases of ultrasonographic interest can be classified into three groups:

- Inflammatory diseases
- Neoplastic diseases
- Obstructive diseases.

The classic inflammatory bowel diseases are uncomplicated acute enteropathy, complicated acute enteropathy and chronic enteropathy.

ULTRASONOGRAPHY IN ENTEROPATHY

Ultrasonography is increasingly popular to study acute and chronic enteropathies, as it allows for evaluating both the system morphology and functionality, and all that in real-time.

ACUTE ENTEROPATHIES

They include **uncomplicated and complicated** acute enteropathies.
   Uncomplicated acute forms:

- The patient may experience a severe symptomatology even with a 'mild' ultrasonographic picture. The ultrasonographic evaluation of the intestinal motility is a key element in these diseases, as symptomatology persists until the small intestine motility is not restored
- Changes concern the lumen content and the motility, without morphological changes of the intestinal wall
- Mild dilation and distension of intestinal loops is observed, with content most fluid than the norm, no tendency to improvement, and/or a gaseous pattern (secondary to the loops hypomotility).

Complicated acute forms: with intestinal perforation, severe changes of parietal stratigraphy and peritoneum involvement are often associated.

BOWEL PERFORATIONS (Fig. 11.11–12)

Diagnosing an intestinal perforation on ultrasonography is not easy, since the wall discontinuity is rarely seen.
Ultrasonographic findings:

- Loss of normal stratigraphy, focal changes (secondary to inflammation), with possible thickening of the area
- **Secondary ultrasonographic signs** are very important and must raise a suspicion of intestinal perforation (they are listed in order of importance and prevalence):
  - Mesentery focal hyperechogenicity with distal echoes dispersion (indicative of focal peritonitis): often, the maximum reaction area around the perforated loop has a crescent shape (Fig. 11.11)
  - Peritoneal effusion (often mild or moderate, with echoic suspended particles)
  - Free abdominal air. To detect a mild-degree pneumoperitoneum, it is recommended to place the

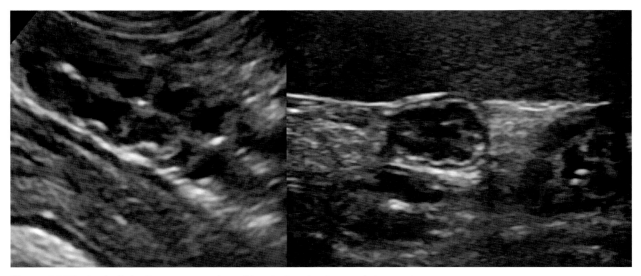

Figure 11.12 Longitudinal and transverse scan of a small intestine loop that shows marked corrugation.

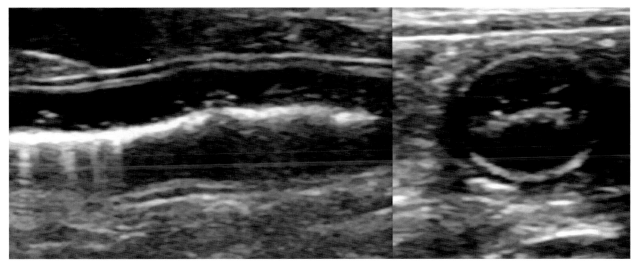

Figure 11.13 Hyperechoic foci in the mucous coat of a patient on an empty stomach.

patient in the right lateral recumbency and hold the probe on the left flank over the splenic body, so there are no interposed intestinal loops that could be misleading. Comet tail or reverberation artefacts, typical of small air collections, are to be searched for (Fig. 11.11).

Other important but less specific ultrasonographic signs:

- Reactivity of regional lymph nodes
- Reduced motility of the gastrointestinal tract
- Intestinal corrugation (Fig. 11.12). Intestinal corrugation is an aspecific ultrasonographic sign, which can also be found in pancreatitis, peritonitis, enteritis, diffuse peritoneal neoplasm, intestinal ischaemia, and acute renal failure.

CHRONIC ENTEROPATHIES IN DOGS
(Fig. 11.13–17)

Patients must definitely be on an empty stomach. Based on a series of studies conducted by Lorrie Gaschen et al. (2008) in

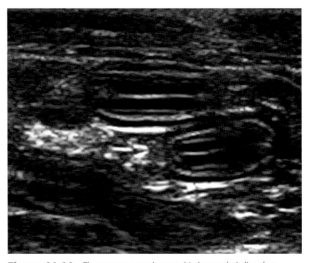

Figure 11.14 The mucous coat shows a thin hyperechoic line that is parallel to the submucosa and to the mucous coat–lumen interface. It is considered a fibrotic reaction of the villous base.

dogs, some correlation was demonstrated between the ultra-sonographic appearance of the GI tract and the response to therapy.

Study results suggest classifying dogs with chronic enteropathy into three groups:

- **Food Responsive (FR):** patients suffering from chronic gastrointestinal symptoms that respond to a dietary therapy,
- **Steroid Responsive (SR):** patients suffering from conditions that respond to steroids,

- **Protein-Losing Enteropathies (PLE):** patients suffering from lymphangiectasia and protein-losing enteropathy.

This approach provides for an ultrasonographic examination carried out after the patient preparation that includes deworming and a one-month hypoallergenic diet.

The ultrasonographic examination is part of a broader context, where lab tests have ruled out contributory conditions. Table 11.3 shows the ultrasonographic differences between these three classes.

TABLE 11.3
Ultrasonographic signs detectable in chronic enteropathies (classification suggested by Gaschen et al. 2008)

	FR	SR	PLE
Content	Normal or slightly fluid	Small collections of food material, too much fluid, which stagnates in loops	Many small intestine loops contain ingesta with a fluid consistency, that stagnates and tends to create tympanism
Mucous coat	Normal or showing small focal changes in echogenicity or echoic foci	1. Hyperechoic foci of the mucous coat (Fig. 11.13)[1] 2. Very thin hyperechoic line within the mucous coat, parallel to the submucosa (Fig. 11.14)[2]	Thickened; often, severe changes in echogenicity: hyperechoic or showing stripes perpendicular to the submucosa, especially in the jejunum (Fig. 11.17)
Submucosa	Normal or slightly thickened	Mild, moderate or severe thickening; sometimes split in two (Fig. 11.15)	Moderate or severe thickening; sometimes split in two
Muscular coat	Normal or mild thickening	Can be thickened (Fig. 11.16)[3]	Often thickened[3]
Motility	From normal to slightly spastic, or moderately reduced	Often reduced	Severe change, from very strong and spastic to absent
Elasticity[4]	Normal	Reduced in some areas	Often very reduced
Lymph nodes	Normal or mild reactivity of jejunal or right colic lymph nodes	Often enlarged or hypoechoic, or too much contrasted compared to surrounding mesentery, due to its hyperechogenicity. Persistent oval shape and hilar vascularization	Variable and not correlated with disease severity

[1] Two different aetiologies are possible:
    a) air micro-bubbles trapped between the villi, with mucous coat hypoplasia;
    b) persistent dilation of lymph nodes.
    Differentiating the two abnormal conditions is not always possible. In case of villous atrophy, mild reduction within the mucous coat can be observed. Often, with lymph nodes dilation, an irregular but diffuse wall hyperechogenicity is often associated. Echoic foci within the mucous coat are a normal finding in patients that were not fasting.
[2] According to the literature, this is a fibrotic band that forms at the villous base. There are contrasting opinions about the possible reversibility of this sign.
[3] It is considered secondary to a chronic spasm of gastrointestinal tract.
[4] The GI tract elasticity is evaluated like this:
    a) in cross section, loops must appear as a classic 'smile' and not corrugated or ovalized;
    b) during peristalsis, wall movements must be symmetrical and synchronized.

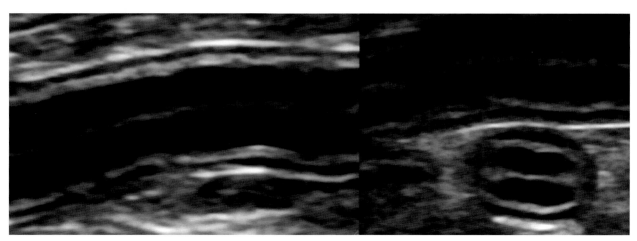

Figure 11.15 Intestinal loop with submucosa thickening.

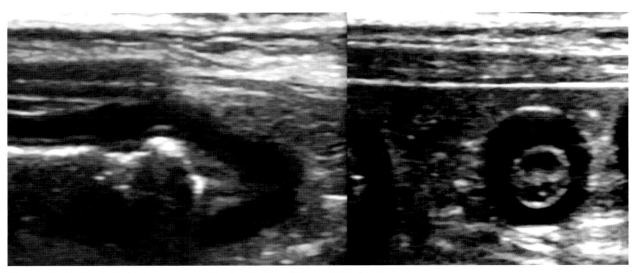

Figure 11.16 Longitudinal and transverse scan of an intestinal loop with severe thickening of muscular coat.

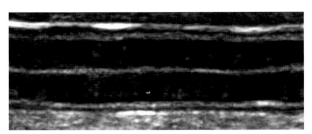

Figure 11.17 The mucous coat shows fine hyperechoic stripes perpendicular to the submucosa. This finding is characteristic of a lymphangiectasia.

CHRONIC ENTEROPATHY IN CATS (Fig. 11.18)

Ultrasonographic signs studied and evaluated in dogs are commonly found in cats too; so, the classification adopted by Gaschen and Kircher was transferred to this species.

In cats, the role of **right colic lymph nodes** is very important. In chronic enteropathies, they are often hypoechoic, rounded, basically dilated, with hyperechoic surrounding mesentery. Asymptomatic patients with these features must raise a suspicion of chronic enteropathy.

Increasingly common are reports of **typhlitis**, detectable on ultrasonography as a cecum focal thickening, associated with loss of normal parietal stratigraphy and reactivity of right colic lymph nodes.

It is very difficult to differentiate a feline chronic **enteropathy** from a **diffuse intestinal lymphoma**: ultrasonographic signs and symptomatology are identical.

Zwingenberger suggests that old cats, with significant thickening of the muscular coat, have a higher risk of diffuse lymphoma rather than inflammatory bowel disease. Not all authors agree.

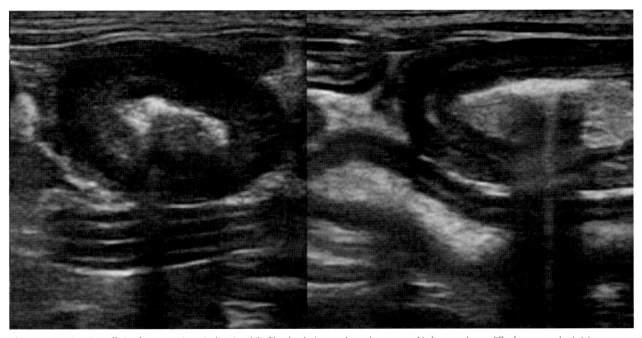

Figure 11.18 Cat suffering from gastrointestinal eosinophilic fibrodysplasia: note how ultrasonographic features do not differ from a neoplastic injury.

Another emerging feline disease that must be recognized and differentiated from an intestinal neoplasm is the gastrointestinal **eosinophilic sclerosing fibroplasia**. It is a symmetrical and concentric injury that changes the parietal stratigraphy and creates intestinal obstructions. It must be differentiated from an intestinal neoplasm (Fig. 11.18).

INTESTINAL NEOPLASMS (Fig. 11.19)

The most often reported neoplasms in the literature in dogs and cats are adenocarcinoma, lymphoma and leiomyosarcoma (Table 11.4) (Fig. 11.19).

Clearly, many other neoplastic diseases can affect the enteric tract.

The next table summarizes the main ultrasonographic features.

It highlights that ultrasonographic findings are often overlapping, especially between adenocarcinoma and intestinal lymphoma. The leiomyosarcoma has slightly different ultrasonographic features. Definitive diagnosis always requires a biopsy.

HOW TO DIFFERENTIATE INTESTINAL NEOPLASMS FROM CHRONIC ENTEROPATHIES

Differentiating a chronic or acute enteropathy from a neoplasm can be difficult.

The literature (Penninck 2003) suggests considering the following ultrasonographic parameters:

Parameter	Neoplasm	Enteropathy
Mean thickness of intestinal wall	1.5 cm	0.6 cm
Parietal stratigraphy	Changed in 99% of patients	Normal in 88% of patients
Number of injuries	Only multifocal in 2% of cases	Two tracts affected at least in 72% of cases
Mean thickness of tributary lymph nodes	1.9 cm	1.0 cm

A single injury that changes the stratigraphy of the intestinal wall has a probability of 50:1 of being an intestinal neoplasm rather than enteritis.

Definitive diagnosis always requires a cytological and histological examination.

OBSTRUCTIVE DISEASES

These diseases cause an occlusion of the intestinal lumen, or stop the advance of food content. Apart from paralytic ileus, they very often require urgent surgery.

TABLE 11.4 Features of the most common intestinal neoplasms		
Intestinal adenocarcinoma	**Intestinal lymphosarcoma**	**Leiomyosarcoma**
Symmetrical and concentric mass	Symmetrical and concentric mass	Asymmetric and eccentric mass
Generally, it is no more than 3.5 cm in length	Generally, it is more than 3.5 cm in length	Generally, it is more than 3.5 cm in length and often has a diameter greater than 3 cm
Changed intestinal stratigraphy	Changed intestinal stratigraphy	Changed intestinal stratigraphy
Often associated with obstructive mechanical ileus	It can cause obstructive mechanical ileus, although more time is needed	Hardly ever causes intestinal obstruction
Regional lymph nodes are very often involved	Regional lymph nodes are often involved	Regional lymph nodes are hardly ever involved
Possibly associated with ulcers	Possibly associated with ulcers	Hardly ever associated with ulcers

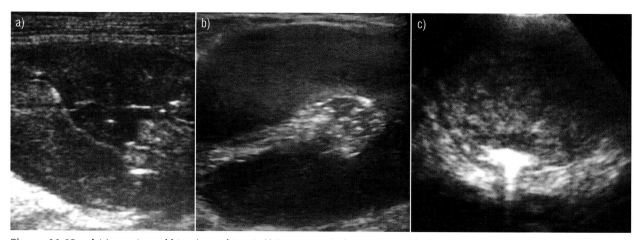

Figure 11.19 a) Adenocarcinoma. **b)** Lymphoma. **c)** Intestinal leiomyosarcoma in three canine patients. There are no pathognomonic elements, and a biopsy is always required to issue a final diagnosis.

FUNCTIONAL OR PARALYTIC ILEUM

This is a paralysis of intestinal peristalsis that affects the whole intestine; it is not caused by an intestinal obstruction but is secondary to several acute abdominal diseases (such as parvovirosis, acute abdomen, abdominal pain, postoperative stasis, vascular damage). Paralytic ileus must be differentiated from mechanical ileus that is due to a mechanical occlusion and requires urgent surgical treatment. Ultrasonographic findings:

- All intestinal loops appear moderately (not severely) dilated
- The gastrointestinal contents is almost always fluid or gaseous
- The motility is often diminished or even absent, with the ingested material swaying back and forth instead of progressing
- Often, the colon is affected to the same extent as the small intestine
- In severe cases, mucous coat hyperechogenicity (especially duodenum and jejunum) is observed, due to accumulation of mucus, cellular debris, proteins and fibrin.

TYPES OF MECHANICAL ILEUS

A mechanical ileus is an intestinal obstruction due to a physical obstacle.

MESENTERIC VOLVULUS (Fig. 11.20)

- The mesenteric volvulus is a rare but very serious disease where one intestinal loop rotates on its own transverse axis or mesenteric axis (unlike the intestinal torsion where the intestine rotates on its own longitudinal axis). Predisposing factors are the breed (German shepherd and Pointer) and a previous gastropexy.
- There are no radiographic or ultrasonographic pathognomonic findings.
- Secondary ultrasonographic signs that head towards this diagnosis are:
  - Some small intestine loops are enormously distended by gas and fluid, while others are empty. It can be difficult to differentiate a small intestine loop from the large intestine, because the loop is very dilated and the wall appears thinned. The dilated loop must be followed until the connection point with the large intestine is identified
  - No foreign bodies or other causes of obstruction are visualized
  - Abnormal **stratigraphy** of the intestinal contents is often visible, with the more dense material deposited as a sediment and the more fluid material forming the supernatant (Fig. 11.20)
  - The wall seems exfoliating within the intestinal lumen
  - If the patient is not seriously polypnoic, the vascularization of affected intestinal loops, which is greatly reduced, can be assessed by Doppler.
- Ultrasonography allows for the serial evaluation of the patient.

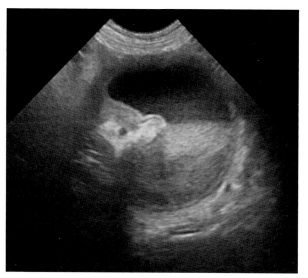

Figure 11.20   Intestinal volvulus in a six-year-old male German shepherd. There are no pathognomonic ultrasonographic signs, but one dilated and hypomobile small intestine loop with plain stratigraphy of endoluminal material must be considered a sign of serious intestinal stasis and indicative of mechanical ileus, especially if intestinal loops are completely normal.

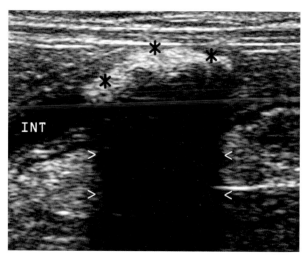

Figure 11.21   Foreign body occluding a patient duodenum. The foreign body was a peach pit. Note the duodenum containing anechoic material, the foreign body hyperechoic interface (*), and the clean posterior shadowing it created (> <).

OCCLUDING FOREIGN BODY (Fig. 11.21)

- The foreign body (FB) appears as a structure with a highly reflective surface, which produces a clean posterior acoustic shadow (Fig. 11.21)
- Intestinal loops upstream of the obstruction are very stretched by fluid and some gas
- Downstream of the occlusion, loops are normal sized, do not contain ingesta and maintain a normal peristalsis
- Dilated loops are followed up to the foreign body and over, so as to verify effective occlusion and possible location

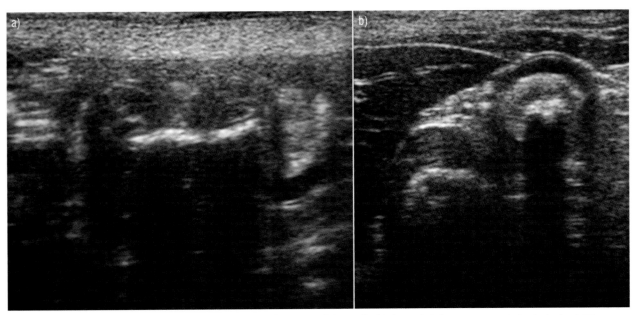

Figure 11.22 Linear foreign body. **a)** Longitudinal scan: intestinal loops are rolled up and a thin hyperechoic line generates posterior shadowing. **b)** Cross-section: a small hyperechoic dot-like structure generates posterior shadowing. If the linear structure is very thin, the posterior shadowing can only be visible in the transverse scan.

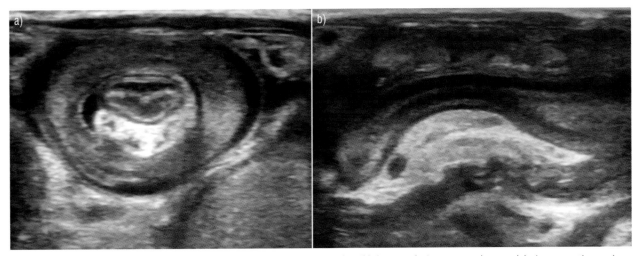

Figure 11.23 **a)** Transverse appearance of an intussusception. The anechoic triangle visible between the intussuscepted tract and the intussuscepting one is a haematoma. When present, it indicates a vascular complication. **b)** Longitudinal or hay fork-like appearance.

- The distension of upstream intestinal loops may be missing if the occlusion involves the proximal intestine and in case of vomiting.

LINEAR FOREIGN BODY (Fig. 11.22)

- As the foreign body is very small, secondary ultrasonographic signs are minimal
- An asymmetrical bowel corrugation is observed
- In the longitudinal scan, a solid hyperechoic line is observed, corresponding to the FB contained in the lumen of intestinal loops asymmetrically piled (Fig. 11.22a)
- In the transverse scan, the hyperechoic line becomes a hyperechoic dot, able to generate clean shadowing (Fig. 11.22b).

INTUSSUSCEPTION (Fig. 11.23)

Intestinal intussusception is produced by the invagination of an intestinal tract into another tract and has very characteristic ultrasonographic appearance:

- In the transverse scan, hypoechoic and hyperechoic rings follow each other concentrically (appearance described as 'concentric rings' or 'bull's eye') (Fig. 11.23a)
- Anechoic outer ring (intussuscepting) created by the overlapping of two intestinal walls folded on themselves. Parietal oedema cancels normal stratigraphy and often makes these loops completely anechoic
  Hyperechoic intermediate ring with variable distal echoes dispersion, depending on the inflammation level (corresponding to the mesentery portion trapped between intestinal loops)

- On the inside the intussuscepted intestinal loop is positioned, maintaining a normal intestinal stratigraphy
- In the longitudinal scan, the intussuscepted loop is contained within the intussuscepting one. This configuration has been called hay fork-like (Fig. 11.23b)
- Sometimes the ileocecocolic valve can mimic an intussusception, especially in the transverse scan. The longitudinal scan is different and allows for an easy distinction.

RECOMMENDED READING

Penninck DG, Smyers B, Webster CR, Rand W, Moore AS: Diagnostic value of ultrasonography in differentiating enteritis from intestinal neoplasia in dogs. Veterinary Radiology & Ultrasound, 2003. 44(5): 570–575.

Gaschen L, Kircher P, Stussi A, Allenspach K, Gaschen F, De Heer M, Grone A: Comparison of ultrasonographic findings with clinical activity index (CIBDAI) and diagnosis in dogs with chronic enteropathies. Veterinary Radiology & Ultrasound, 2008, 49(1): 56–64.

Stander N, Wagner WM, Goddard A, Kirberger RM: Normal canine pediatric gastrointestinal ultrasonography. Vet Rad & Ultrasound, 2010, 51(1), p 75–78.

Craig LE, Hardam EE, Hertzke DM, Flatland B, Rohrbach BW, Moore RR: Feline gastrointestinal eosinophilic sclerosing fibroplasia. Vet Pathol, 2009, 46: 63–70.

Zwingenberger AL, Marks SL, Baker TW and Moore PF: Ultrasonographic evaluation of the muscolaris propria in cats with diffuse small intestinal lymphoma or inflammatory bowel disease. J Vet Intern Med, 2010, 24, p 289–292.

12 Pancreas ultrasonography

Edoardo Auriemma

SCAN TECHNIQUE (Fig. 12.1–4)

Animal preparation	• 12 hours on an empty stomach, at least. • Wide hair-clipping, including intercostal spaces. • Dorsal recumbency, right and left lateral.
Probes	• Microconvex, 5 MHz mean frequency (3–8 MHz). • Linear, high-frequency (7.5–12 MHz), for small breed animals and organ superficial portions.
Scans and respective probe position (Fig. 12.1, 12.2, 12.3) 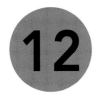	• **Left lobe: longitudinal and transverse scan (position 5).** Starting at position 7, the probe is moved along the edge of the left costal arch, remaining as perpendicular as possible to the patient's skin surface. Only a very light pressure on the probe is needed. The probe travel ends as far as a triangular region between the stomach fundus cranially, the spleen superficially, and the left kidney caudolaterally (position 5) is identified (Fig. 12.1a). After having visualized the extraparenchymal portion of the splenic vein, try to follow its course up to its outlet into the portal vein. Typically, the outlet takes place towards the centre of the abdomen, slightly to the left, when the portal vein deviates ventrally and to the right, and receives the splenic vein. The outlet of the splenic vein, that goes from the body (central abdomen) to the left lobe (left abdomen), is the vascular landmark to visualize the pancreas left lobe (Fig. 12.2). Sometimes, and most clearly in cats, in the central portion of the pancreas left lobe the pancreatic duct can be visualized as a tubular structure of 0.5–2 mm in diameter with anechoic centre and hyperechoic walls. • **Body: longitudinal and oblique scan (position 7–8).** Place the probe caudally to the xyphoid process with the beam longitudinally oriented, starting from a median-paramedian right position. Tilt the probe until the prehilar portion of the portal vein is visualized (Fig. 12.1b). The pancreas body is located caudally to the stomach (caudodorsally to the pyloric region) and ventrally to the portal vein (Fig. 12.3). • **Right lobe: longitudinal and intercostal scan (positions 8 and 8').** With the probe caudal to the right costal arch and the beam longitudinally oriented, scan the region that goes from the right kidney, caudally, to the pyloric-duodenal junction (Fig. 12.1c). The proximal duodenum as a landmark may be helpful (see Chapter 11, p. 101). After having identified the duodenum, a transverse scan of this organ is performed trying to identify the pancreaticoduodenal vein, which runs to the centre of the pancreatic parenchyma (Fig. 12.4). After having identified the pancreas right lobe, transverse and longitudinal scans are performed. In deep-chested dogs, the right intercostal approach is useful, keeping the probe perpendicular to the rib cage, about half the ribs' length. Move cranially up to identify the liver visceral edge. After having identified this edge, it is followed starting as dorsally as possible until the duodenum is identified.

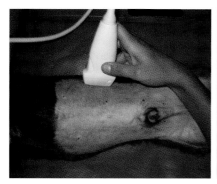

Figure 12.1a Position 5. The left pancreatic lobe is identified within the triangle formed by the stomach, spleen and kidney. The splenic vein and portal vein are important anatomical landmarks.

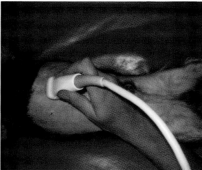

Figure 12.1b Position 7. Just caudally to the body of the stomach the body of the pancreas is located.

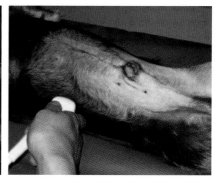

Figure 12.1c Position 8. The pancreas right lobe is next to the proximal duodenum; the intercostal approach is often preferable, especially in deep-chested dogs.

ULTRASONOGRAPHIC ANATOMY

Location	Cranial abdomen: middle, right and left.
Morphology	• **Three regions**: right lobe, body and left lobe. In dogs, the most commonly identifiable and developed is the right lobe. In cats, the more developed pancreatic lobe is the left lobe, which features a hook-like ending. In geriatric cats finding a partial dilation of the pancreatic duct is common. • Elongated inverted-V shape, directed cranially.

Relationships with adjacent organs evaluable on ultrasonography	• **Right lobe**
	  – **Cranially**: pyloric-duodenal junction.
	  – **Ventrolaterally**: descending duodenum.
	  – **Dorsally**: right kidney.
	  – **Vascular landmark**: gastroduodenal vein that runs in the pancreatic parenchyma of the right lobe.
	• **Body**
	  – **Cranially**: pyloric-duodenal junction, body of the stomach.
	  – **Vascular landmark**: portal vein, located dorsally to the pancreas body.
	• **Left lobe**
	  – **Cranially**: gastric body and fundus.
	  – **Laterally**: spleen.
	  – **Caudolaterally**: left kidney.
	• Vascular landmark: splenic vein.

Echogenicity	• Isoechoic compared to surrounding fat. • Isoechoic: slightly hyperechoic compared to the liver. • Hypoechoic compared to surrounding mesentery in the puppy, so more easily identifiable.
Echostructure	• Homogeneous.
Tributary lymph nodes	• **Gastric, gastroduodenal.** • **Hepatic.** • **Splenic.** • **Mesenteric.**

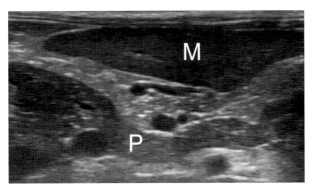

Figure 12.2 Pancreatic left lobe in a cat; the anechoic circular structure in contact with the pancreas to the left of the image is the portal vein.

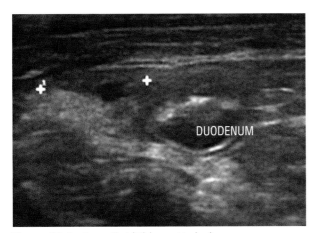

Figure 12.3 The pancreatic body is delimited by the stomach and the portal vein (down and on the left).

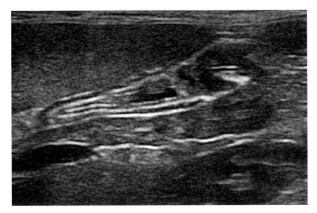

Figure 12.4 Pancreatic right lobe, next to duodenum.

ULTRASONOGRAPHIC CHANGES: PANCREATIC DISEASES

Most common pancreatic diseases of ultrasonographic interest can be classified into three groups:

- Inflammatory diseases
- Neoplastic diseases
- Miscellaneous diseases.

The ultrasonographic examination must be systematic.

INFLAMMATORY DISEASES: PANCREATITIS (Fig. 12.5–8)

The sensitivity of ultrasonographic examination in the diagnosis of pancreatitis varies depending on the species (a dog is different from a cat) and whether the disease is acute or chronic. Especially in cats, sensitivity is particularly low; so, this disease cannot be diagnosed on the sole ultrasonographic picture, but must be correlated with the patient's clinical and haematological examination. Consequently, when pancreatitis is clinically suspected, despite the ultrasonographic examination not being conclusive for a pancreatic disease, this cannot, be excluded.

Ultrasonographic findings that are consistent and more often associated with acute pancreatitis in dogs and cats include:

- Enlarged pancreas, often focally (many cases of pancreatitis affecting one or two pancreas portions, not the whole organ)
- Irregular echostructure and heterogeneous echogenicity, mainly hypoechoic (Fig. 12.5)

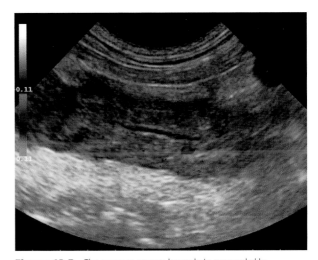

Figure 12.5 The pancreas appears hypoechoic, surrounded by hyperechoic mesentery, with distal echoes dispersion and greatly enlarged. These findings are typical of acute pancreatitis. In this patient, the whole pancreatic lobe is affected by the process.

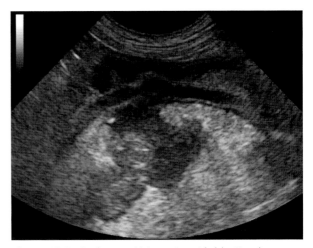

Figure 12.6 Focal pancreatitis in a patient; right lobe. Note the same characteristics of Figure 12.5; however, in this case pancreatitis is not extended to the whole lobe. The surrounding mesentery is hyperechoic, with distal echoes dispersion.

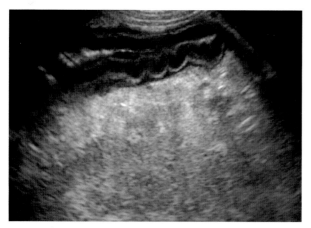

Figure 12.7 The duodenal corrugation associated to hyperechoic mesentery with distal echoes dispersion is a typical aspect of pancreatitis.

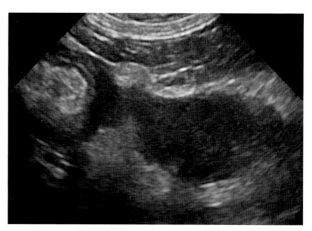

Figure 12.9 Hypoechoic pancreatic mass with irregular edges, associated with distal echoes dispersion (pancreatic adenocarcinoma).

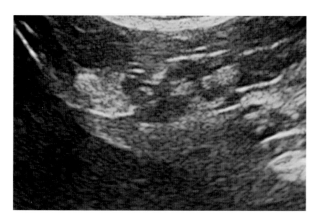

Figure 12.8 Changes in echostructure, hyperechogenicity and shape, not associated with increased pancreas volume or distal echoes dispersion by surrounding tissues: chronic pancreatitis.

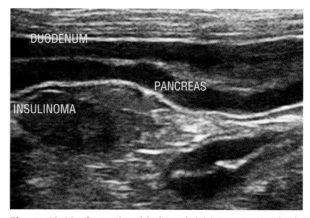

Figure 12.10 Pancreatic nodular hypoechoic injury not associated with distal echoes dispersion (insulinoma).

- Hyperechoic peripancreatic fat (peripancreatic steatitis) with distal echoes dispersion (Fig. 12.6)
- Peripancreatic effusion or ascites (less frequently)
- Often, duodenum parietal thickening is associated, which may have a 'corrugated, accordion-like' appearance (Fig. 12.7) or show signs of paralytic ileus (hypomotility with content fluid pattern)
- Possible extrahepatic cholestasis especially in cats.

Ultrasonographic findings associated with a **chronic pancreatitis** in dogs and cats include:

- Not enlarged pancreas
- Mostly irregular edges
- Irregular echostructure and heterogeneous echogenicity, with hyperechoic areas that feature irregular edges and are not associated with distal echoes dispersion in the pancreatic parenchyma (Fig. 12.8)
- Sometimes, hyperechogenicity of the peripancreatic fat not associated with distal echoes dispersion, consistent with chronic peripancreatic steatitis.

NEOPLASTIC DISEASES (Fig. 12.9–10)

Most frequent pancreatic neoplasms in dogs and cats are epithelial neoplasms of exocrine (adenocarcinoma, carcinoma) and endocrine (insulinomas) portions.

From an ultrasonographic point of view, pancreatic adenocarcinomas are often not clearly distinguishable from a pancreatitis; so, correlating ultrasonographic signs with the patient clinical examination and confirming the suspected diagnosis by cytology are essential.

Ultrasonographic findings consistent with exocrine pancreatic neoplasms (adenocarcinomas/carcinomas) are:

- Hypoechoic masses with a complex or mixed echogenicity (Fig. 12.9)
- Poorly defined, blurred or irregular edges
- Often associated to the inflammation of the surrounding pancreatic parenchyma; this is why they are not always distinguishable from an ultrasonographic picture of pancreatitis
- Often, they metastasize to other organs (liver, regional lymph nodes)
- Tributary adenopathy.

The diagnosis of insulinoma is based on clinical symptoms and laboratory tests (hypoglycaemia associated with hyperinsulinemia). The ultrasonographic examination may help the clinician to manage the patient. There are two main forms of insulinoma: the miliary form where no ultrasound detectable very small nodules infiltrate the pancreas, and the nodular form (well-defined nodules identifiable on ultrasonography). If the patient is suffering from single nodules, it could be a surgical candidate. Unfortunately, the ultrasonography is disappointing in identifying metastases, both in pancreatic lymph nodes (their position along the course of the proximal duodenum varies; moreover, to differentiate a primary insulinoma from lymph node metastases in the right pancreatic lobe is often hard due to the contiguity of these organs), and in the liver, because almost always metastatic liver nodules are isoechoic compared to the surrounding parenchyma due to an insulinoma. To date, the gold standard to stage these patients is the CT examination, but ultrasonography is widely used as a screening.

Ultrasonographic findings are consistent with endocrine pancreatic neoplasms.

- Nodular rounded neoformations, which partly change the pancreatic anatomy (Fig. 12.10)
- They have a mass effect and divert pancreatic vessels
- Well-defined edges
- Predominantly hypoechoic with homogeneous echostructure
- Often, they metastasize to other organs (liver, regional lymph nodes)
- Tributary adenopathy.

MISCELLANEOUS DISEASES
The following pancreatic changes fall into this subclass:

- Nodular hyperplasia
- Cavitary injuries (cysts, pseudocysts, abscesses)
- Pancreatic oedema.

NODULAR HYPERPLASIA (Fig. 12.11)
Nodular pancreatic lesions without a neoplastic nature (nodular hyperplasia) have been described in both dogs and older cats; when injuries are single and focal, it is impossible to differentiate this condition from pancreatic neoplasms based only on ultrasonographic examination and the diagnosis must be cytologically confirmed (Fig. 12.9) Often, nodular hyperplastic injuries are multiple, well-defined and scattered in the pancreatic parenchyma; moreover, the patient is asymptomatic and blood sugar is within normal limits.

Ultrasonographic findings:

- Multiple isoechoic or hypoechoic nodules with a homogeneous echostructure
- Well-defined edges (Fig. 12.11)
- The pancreas is rarely enlarged
- Peripancreatic tissues are normal

CAVITARY INJURIES (Fig. 12.12–13)
The most common cavitary injuries with a fluid content include cysts, pseudocysts and abscesses. Pancreatic cysts and pseudocysts (Fig. 12.12) are secondary to past pancreatitis events that caused parenchymal necrosis areas. Based on the sole ultrasonographic examination it is not possible to differentiate a cyst from an abscess (Fig. 12.13) or from a cavitary neoplasm: in these cases the clinical examination, the cytology of injuries and an ultrasonographic follow-up are essential to achieve a correct ultrasonographic diagnosis.

Ultrasonographic findings:

- Round structures with more or less defined edges and posterior-wall enhancement areas (fluid content)
- A content that is basically more anechoic in cysts and more echoic in abscesses, even if mixed forms are frequent

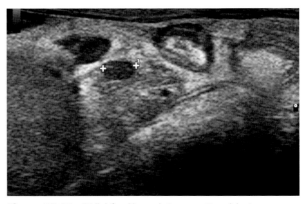

Figure 12.11 Well-defined hypoechoic pancreatic nodules in a pancreas otherwise within normal limits, in an asymptomatic patient with normal blood sugar (nodular hyperplasia).

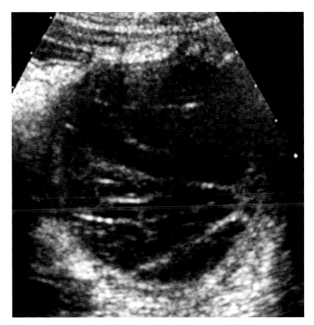

Figure 12.12 Anechoic injury, with echoic septa and fluid contents. Cytologically, this injury turned out to be a pancreatic pseudocyst, but you cannot differentiate it from a pancreatic septate abscess on ultrasonography.

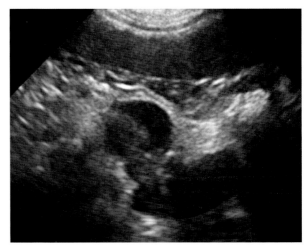

Figure 12.13 Heterogeneous cavitary injury of the left pancreatic lobe. This cavity turned out to be an abscess.

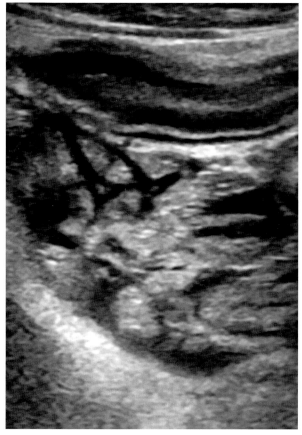

Figure 12.13 Pancreatic enlargement with heterogeneous echostructure and 'striped' appearance (pancreatic oedema).

- Possible multilocular septate appearance (pseudocysts, abscesses).

PANCREATIC OEDEMA (Fig. 12.14)

The pancreatitis should not be confused on ultrasonography with the pancreatic oedema which may be associated with an inflammatory disease of the pancreas, but more often is secondary to other disease conditions, such as hypoproteinemia and portal hypertension. In cases of pancreatic oedema, the pancreas has a distinctive 'striped' appearance with predominantly parallel hypoechoic septa which run in its parenchyma.

Ultrasonographic findings:

- Increased pancreatic volume
- Hyperechoic peripancreatic fat
- Hyperechoic parenchyma crossed by hypoechoic stripes
- Sometimes, the organ can be delimited by a mild effusion.

RECOMMENDED READING

Anderson et al. Pancreatic abscess in 36 dogs: a retrospective analysis of prognostic indicators. JAAHA. 2008, 44(4) 171–179.

Hecht S, Henry G: Sonographic Evaluation of the Normal and Abnormal Pancreas. Clinical Techniques in Small Animal Practice. 2007, 22(3): 115–121.

Zoran DL: Pancreatitis in cats: diagnosis and management of a challenging disease. Journal of the American Animal Hospital Association. 2006, 42(1): 1–9.

Saunders HM, VanWinkle T.J, Drobatz K, Kimmel SE, Washabau RJ: Ultrasonographic findings in cats with clinical, gross pathologic, and histologic evidence of acute pancreatic necrosis: 20 cases (1994–2001). Journal of the American Veterinary Medical Association. 2002, 221(12): 1724–1730.

VanEnkevort BA, O'Brien RT, Young KM: Pancreatic pseudocyst in 4 dogs and 2 cats: ultrasonographic and clinicopathologic findings. J Vet Intern Med. 1999 Jul-Aug; 13(4): 309–313.

Lamb CR: Pancreatic edema in dogs with hypoalbuminemia or portal hypertension. JVIM. 1999, 13: 498–500.

Hess RS, Saunders HM, Van Winkle TJ, Shofer FS, Washabau RJ: Clinical, clinicopathologic, radiographic, and ultrasonographic abnormalities in dogs with fatal acute pancreatitis: 70 cases (1986–1995).

Journal of the American Veterinary Medical Association. 1998, 23(5): 665–670.

Female reproductive system

Giliola Spattini

SCAN TECHNIQUE (Fig. 13.1)

Animal preparation	• 12 hours on an empty stomach, at least. • Wide hair-clipping of the middle-caudal abdomen flanks included. • Dorsal recumbency, right and/or left lateral, standing animal.
Probes	• Microconvex, 7.5 MHz mean frequency. • Linear high-frequency (7.5–10 MHz), especially for the caudal portion of the uterus and uterine horns of medium-small breed animals.

Scans and respective probe position 	• **Uterus:**
	  1. Transverse scan (position 1): The patient is preferably in the right lateral recumbency or the ventrodorsal recumbency. The probe is just cranial to the pubic bone (palpable), over the linea alba (Fig. 13.1a). The tilt is perpendicular to the skin, the beam is transversely oriented. The probe is moved cranially, until you identify the bladder and the colon on the same transverse plane. Select a caudal scan plane, just cranially to the bladder neck. The bladder is the ventral landmark, the colon is the dorsal landmark, iliac arteries are the lateral landmarks. When you identify the body, move the probe cranially until the bifurcation, then follow uterine horns up to the ovaries.
	  2. Longitudinal scan (position 1): after having found the uterine body using the transverse scan, rotate the probe by 90 degrees (Fig. 13.1b). Follow the uterine body until it bifurcates into the two horns. The thickness at this level is minimal, and the image is sharper using the transverse scan. Often, intestinal loops interfere with the visualization of the uterine course, especially if the patient is not on an empty stomach.
	• **Left ovary:**
	  1. Longitudinal scan (position 4): The patient is in the right lateral recumbency. Palpate the caudal profile of the last rib on the left side that is placed dorsally. Place the probe just caudally to the last rib profile, in the more dorsal portion, just ventrally to the lumbar spine (Fig. 13.1c). The probe is perpendicular to the patient's surface. Identify the left kidney and get a longitudinal image of the caudal pole. From this image, move the probe caudally and tilt the tip laterally. The ovary is located in an area bounded anteriorly by the kidney, medially by the abdominal great vessels (aorta and caudal vena cava), dorsally by epaxial muscles and caudoventrally by free loops of the small intestine.
	  2. Transverse scan: from the longitudinal scan, rotate the probe by 90 degrees to obtain a transverse scan of the ovary (Fig. 13.1d).
	• **Right ovary:**
	  1. Longitudinal scan (position 9): The patient in the left lateral recumbency. Palpate the last intercostal space on the right side. Place the probe on the last intercostal space, in the more dorsal portion, just ventrally to the lumbar spine (Fig. 13.1e). Locate the right kidney and get a longitudinal image of the caudal pole. From here, move the probe caudally until you cross the last rib, keeping the caudal pole of the right kidney still in the image, and tilt the probe slightly medially.
	  2. Transverse scan: from the longitudinal scan, rotate the probe by 90 degrees to obtain a transverse scan of the ovary (Fig. 13.1f).

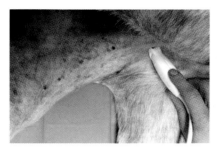

Figure 13.1a Position 1, transverse scan of the corpus uteri.

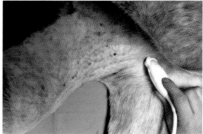

Figure 13.1b Position 1, longitudinal scan of the corpus uteri.

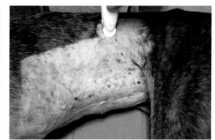

Figure 13.1c Just caudally to position 4, longitudinal scanning of the left ovary.

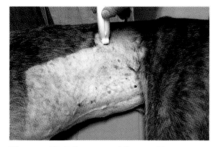

Figure 13.1d Just caudally to position 4, transverse scan of the left ovary.

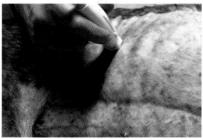

Figure 13.1e Just caudally to position 9, longitudinal scan of the right ovary.

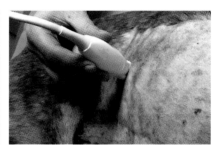

Figure 13.1f Just caudally to position 9, transverse scan of the right ovary.

ULTRASONOGRAPHIC ANATOMY (Fig. 13.2–8)

Localization (Fig. 13.2)	**Uterus:** • Caudal abdomen, left flank and right flank. **Left ovary:** • Left flank. **Right ovary:** • Right flank.
Morphology	**Uterus:** • The uterus during anoestrus or diestrus looks like a tubular small-sized structure, slightly hypoechoic compared to surrounding tissues. Longitudinally, it appears as a hypoechoic regular and well-defined band which tapers further, especially after branching into the two uterine horns (Fig. 13.3). The wall is layered and there is a mucous coat, a muscular coat and a serous coat. They are often not distinguishable and the wall appears uniform. The lumen does not contain any material or includes a thin mucous lining that creates an endoluminal widespread hyperechoic line. The uterine content is never anechoic. • During proestrus and oestrus, the mucous coat can be thickened and more hypoechoic, but the surface remains regular. Often there is an increased hyperechoic endoluminal content (Fig. 13.4). **Ovaries:** • During diestrus and anestrus, the ovary is small-sized and you cannot differentiate any anatomical structures. It appears as a small rounded or oval formation, slightly hypoechoic compared to surrounding tissues (Fig. 13.5). • During proestrus the follicles begin to appear as ill-defined anechoic structures of about 1–2 mm (Fig. 13.6). These structures gradually increase in size, to reach the size of 4–6 mm at the end of proestrus. • During the oestrous, follicular structures are very marked and if they came in great numbers, the organ morphology can change till it resembles a sliced orange. Follicles can reach 10 mm in diameter (Fig. 13.7). • In early stages of the corpus luteum development there is often a certain amount of serohaemorrhagic fluid that makes it similar to an ovulatory follicle (Fig. 13.8). • Around 30 days after the end of oestrus, the ovary regresses to an ill-defined structure that is isoechoic compared to surrounding tissues.

(Continued →)

ULTRASONOGRAPHIC ANATOMY (Continued)

Relationships with adjacent organs evaluable on ultrasonography	**Uterus:** • The bladder is the ventral landmark, the colon is the dorsal landmark, iliac arteries are the lateral landmarks (Fig. 13.2). Select a caudal scan plane, just cranially to the bladder neck. **Left ovary:** • It is located in an area bounded cranially by the left kidney, medially by the abdominal great vessels (aorta and caudal vena cava), dorsally by muscle tissue and caudoventrally by free loops of the small intestine. • From the caudal pole of the kidney, move the probe caudally and tilt the probe tip slightly laterally. **Right ovary:** • It is located in an area bounded cranially by the right kidney, medially by the abdominal great vessels (aorta and caudal vena cava), dorsally by muscle tissue and caudoventrally by free loops of the small intestine. • From the caudal pole of the right kidney, move the probe caudally and tilt it slightly medially. The right ovary is more distant from the caudal pole compared to the right kidney, and often it does not remain in the scan image. It is more medial compared to the left ovary.
Size	**Uterus:** • Transverse diameter in anoestrus (dog e cat): 3–10 mm. • Transverse diameter during oestrus: about 4 mm higher. **Ovaries:** • Longitudinal diameter during anoestrus: dog <20 mm, cat <10 mm. • Ovary volume during oestrus: up to 400% higher than the anoestrus volume.
Edges	**Uterus:** • Thin, smooth and regular. **Ovaries:** • Thin, smooth and regular. Not always clearly distinguishable from surrounding organs, especially during anoestrus. • During oestrous, they are much more defined and easily recognizable.
Echogenicity	**Uterus:** • Hypoechoic compared to the surrounding mesentery; from mildly to markedly hypoechoic depending on the oestrous phase. **Ovaries:** • Hypoechoic compared to the surrounding mesentery; from mildly to markedly hypoechoic depending on the oestrous phase.
Echostructure	**Uterus:** • Mean, basically homogeneous. • In the cervical portion the parietal stratification may be partly recognizable. Ovaries: • Fine during anoestrus. • Non-uniform and coarse during oestrus.
Vessels	**Ovarian veins:** • The left vein ends in the left renal vein; the right vein ends directly in the vena cava caudally, and in the right renal vein ventrally. **Ovarian arteries:** • They originate from the abdominal aorta, caudally and ventrally to the renal arteries.
Tributary lymph nodes	• The main lymphocentre includes the medial iliac lymph nodes (sublumbar), but they also drain in hypogastric and sacral lymph nodes.

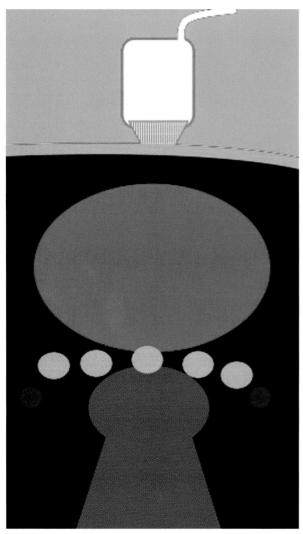

Figure 13.2 Landmarks of the corpus uteri, transverse scan, position 1. Ventrally you see the bladder (yellow), laterally the iliac arteries (red), dorsally the colon (brown). The uterus can take one of these positions (pink dots).

TABLE 13.1 Timing of foetal development	
Days after conception	**foetal development**
10	Uterine vesicles appear (Fig. 13.9)
14	The uterine wall appears layered
16–18	Early outlines of the embryo (Fig. 13.10)
22–24 (18 cat)	Cardiac activity (Fig. 13.11)
27–30	The elongated foetus becomes bipolar and the head is recognizable (Fig. 13.12)
28–31	Limb buds appear
around 29	A fluid-filled stomach is identifiable (Fig. 13.13)
34 (30 cat)	Foetal movements begin
38–42 (29–32 cat)	The liver (hypoechoic) and lungs (hyperechoic) stand out
38–43	Best span of time to sex foetuses
41–43	Foetal kidneys stand out (Fig. 13.14)
around 50	Skeleton bones create a clean acoustic shadow (Fig. 13.15)
around 59	The foetal bowel peristalsis appears
around 60	Initial mineralization of foetal phalanges
around 61	Sealing of the hyaloid artery that nourishes the foetus lens (Fig. 13.16)

Table 13.2 contains other information the ultrasonography can provide about a pregnancy.

ULTRASONOGRAPHIC MEASUREMENTS DURING PREGNANCY (Table 13.3)

Note that the veterinary literature lacks studies using large numbers of pregnancies, and available data relate mostly to Beagle and Labrador retriever bitches. So (adding that the dog shows a high breed variability), the standard deviation of these measurements remains high (more or less than three days), making measurements often useless. In cats there is less variability, but foetal sizes are heavily influenced by the number of foetuses.

PREGNANCY (Fig. 13. 9–22, Tables 13.1 and 13.2)

If the female mates during oestrus, in a healthy subject with a normal reproductive system there is an 87% probability that a pregnancy will start.

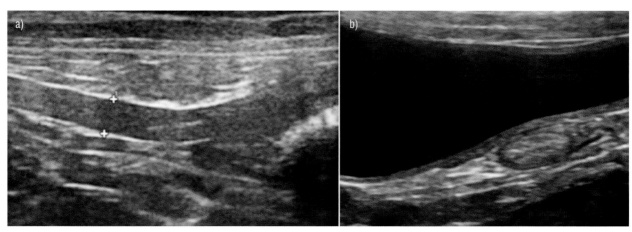

Figure 13.3 a) Longitudinal scan and b) transverse scan of a uterus in anoestrus.

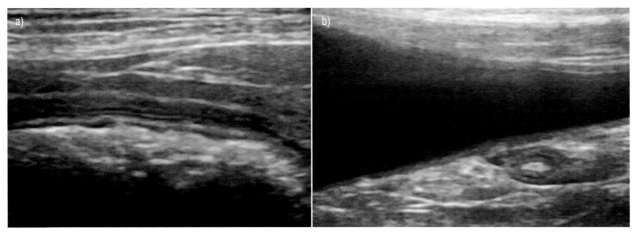

Figure 13.4   a) Longitudinal scan and b) transverse scan of a uterus in oestrus. Note that during oestrus, the uterine wall appears layered and hypoechoic, often showing a thin layer of mucous, then echoic, endoluminal material.

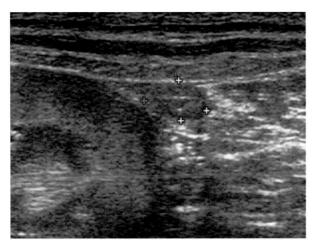

Figure 13.5   Position 4, longitudinal scan of the left ovary during anoestrus.

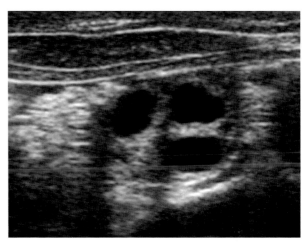

Figure 13.7   Ovary during oestrus: the follicular structures are well-defined and can change the ovarian morphology.

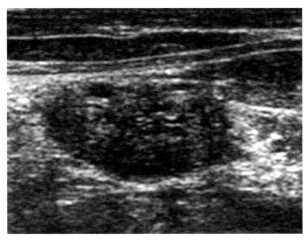

Figure 13.6   Ovary during proestrus: there are very small anechoic structures, scattered in the parenchyma.

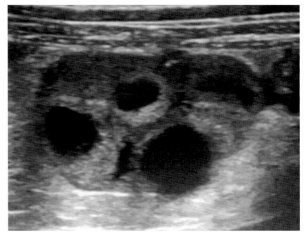

Figure 13.8   The central anechoic collection makes the corpora lutea resemble ovulatory follicles. However, note the shape and thick wall of structures of this ovary and compare them with the preovulatory ovarian follicles in Figure 13.7. Irregular shape and thick wall are typical elements that distinguish a corpus luteum.

TABLE 13.2 Other useful information during pregnancy		
Number of foetuses	It is an unreliable measurement due to the mirror effect (75% accuracy)	Around the 30th day is the best time to state their number
Foetal viability	Foetal heartbeats must be in the 200–240 bpm range (Fig. 13.17) Less than 160 bpm indicates foetal distress Less than 120 bpm indicates high risk of foetal death	Breed variations (hunting dogs show the smaller lower limit)
Foetal resorption	The gestational sac is lost, with accumulation of echoic material in the lumen (Fig. 13.18)	There are no longer any visible foetal structures
Risk factors for a Cesarean section	Lack of uterine fluid. Big-sized skull (Fig. 13.19). Signs of foetal distress. Incomplete cervical plug (Fig. 13.20)	Brachycephalic breeds Puppies' father larger than the mother History of uterine inertia Obesity One or a few foetuses

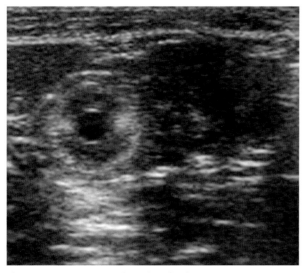

Figure 13.9 Uterine vesicle 10 days after the conception.

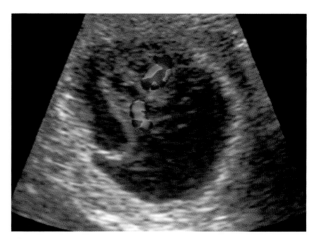

Figure 13.11 Cardiac activity in a foetus, about 23 days after the conception.

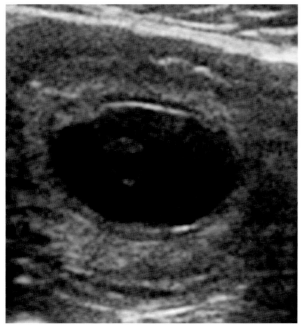

Figure 13.10 Early outlines of the embryo.

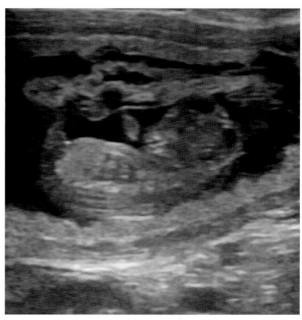

Figure 13.12 The foetus becomes bipolar and the head becomes different from the trunk.

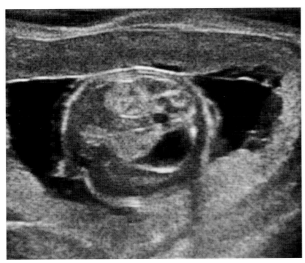

Figure 13.13 The stomach is identifiable as a drop-like structure containing anechoic material.

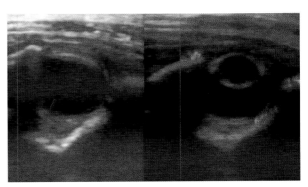

Figure 13.16 a) Foetal eye with a clear circle in the hyaloid artery (red Doppler). b) Foetal eye that does not show the circle in the hyaloid artery. Note that to obtain a Doppler flow from this very fine structure, the eye must be perfectly perpendicular with the primary ultrasound beam.

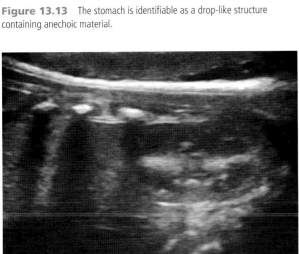

Figure 13.14 The foetal kidney is identifiable.

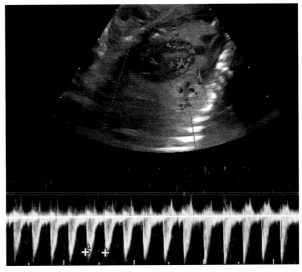

Figure 13.17 PW (Pulsed Wave) Doppler study of the foetal heartbeat.

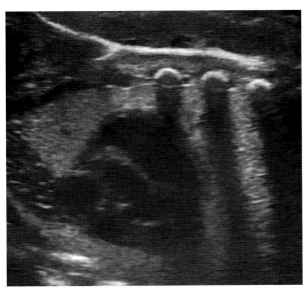

Figure 13.15 The foetal rib creates a strong hyperechoic interface, followed by a clean shadowing.

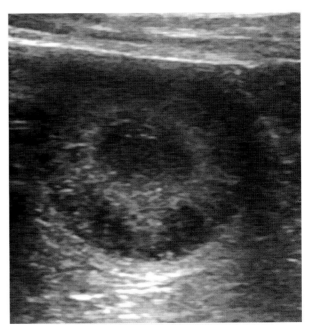

Figure 13.18 Typical ultrasonographic appearance of a foetal resorption.

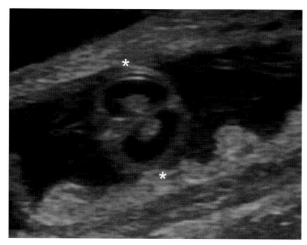

Figure 13.19 Foetal skull diameter: if high, increased risk of Cesarean section. Unfortunately there are no references that can help in defining when a skull is 'too big'. A good method is to perform a lateral and a ventrodorsal radiography of the bitch caudal abdomen and compare the diameter of the birth canal with the size of the foetal skull. This must be at least 5–8 mm less, considering the walls of structures that are normally contained in the pelvic canal.

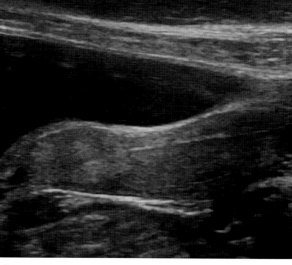

Figure 13.20 Complete uterine cervical plug. If you see anechoic stripes or cavities it is likely that the patient prematurely loses much of the uterine fluid. An excessive reduction in uterine fluid predisposes to a Cesarean section.

Taking all that into account, studying the development of foetal organs together with gathering the clinical information (breast descent, drop in temperature, relaxation of perineal and vaginal tissues) and the history (mating date, progesterone value and oestrus end date), are the most useful elements to schedule a Cesarean section.

Table 13.3 shows the most commonly used measurements and the range of applicability.

TABLE 13.3 Ultrasonographic measurements during pregnancy		
	Literature	**Staff experience**
Dog pregnancy length	63 ±1 day, but can range from 57 to 72 days (Luvoni et al. JSAP 2000)	65 days after the LH peak (when measurable): otherwise 65 days after the serum progesterone reaches 2 ng/ml
	65 ±2 days Lenard et al. Aust Vet J 2007	62 days from the mating day
	65 + 1 days for dogs <9 Kg 65 – 2 days for dogs >40 kg: Kutzler et al. Theriogenology 2003	Delivery expected 57 days after the end of oestrus: typically earlier if there are many puppies, later if there are a few puppies
Cat pregnancy length	63–67 days after the conception Zambelli et al. Theriogenology 2006	Typically, Maine Coons have a pregnancy a few days longer than other breeds
Embryonic vesicle (EV) (Fig. 13.21)	Days before delivery Up to 9 kg: (EV in mm – 82.13 mm)/1.8 From 10 to 25 kg: (EV in mm – 68.68)/1.53 Maltese: 63.2 – (18.58 + 0.71 × EV in mm) Yorkshire: 63.4 – (18.92 + 0.65 × EV in mm) Luvoni et al. Reprod Dom Anim 2006	Useful (even if not very precise) from the 20th to the 40th gestation day, but not in large breed dogs (>25 kg)
	Days after the LH peak: 19.66 + 6.27 × EV in cm Yeager et al. Am J Vet Res 1992	
England's combined formula (Fig. 13.22)	Days before delivery: 34.27 – 5.89 × BD in cm – 2.77 × SBD in cm (BD) = Body Diameter (SBD) = Skull Biparietal Diameter England et al. JSAP 1990 (Labrador)	Usable from the 30th to the 39th day after the LH peak; this window of opportunity is quite accurate but too narrow
SBD (Skull Biparietal Diameter)	Small breed dog (<10 kg): Days before delivery = (SBD in mm – 25.11)/0.61	
	Medium breed dog (<25 kg) Days before delivery = (SBD in mm – 29.18)/0.7 (SBD) = Skull Biparietal Diameter Luvoni et al. JSAP 2000	Usable from the 30th to the 39th day after the LH peak

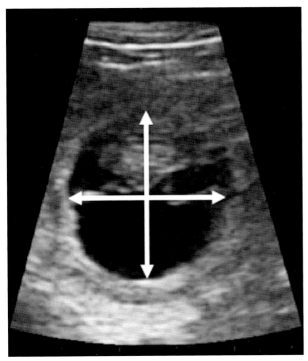

Figure 13.21 EV (EMBRYONIC VESICLE). To obtain this measure, consider the inner diameter of the embryonic vesicle. Since the vesicle tends to be oval, measure the two orthogonal axes, add them up, then take their average. Repeat it for a minimum of three foetuses. Add up these three values and take their average. Put the final value into the formula.

UTERINE DISEASES

The most common uterine diseases of ultrasonographic interest can be classified into three groups:

- Inflammatory diseases
- Endocrine diseases
- Neoplastic diseases.

INFLAMMATORY DISEASES

The most common inflammatory diseases affecting the uterus are endometritis, pyometra, uterine stump disease and uterine torsion.

ENDOMETRITIS (Fig. 13.23)
- The profile of uterine mucous coat is irregular
- There may be small hypoechoic fluid collections
- Typically there is no substantial collection of endoluminal material
- Endometrial cysts are a possible finding (predisposing factor).

PYOMETRA (Fig. 13.24)
- Endoluminal accumulation of purulent fluid material
- The echogenicity can range from anechoic to echoic, and the fluid content is very viscous and rich in echoic floating particles
- The uterine wall can range from normal to irregular and thickened
- There can be hyperechogenicity, with distal echoes dispersion of surrounding tissues
- Not always differentiable from the hydrometra.

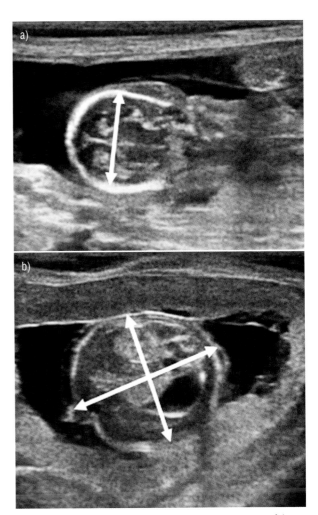

Figure 13.22 England's combined formula: **a)** On a minimum of three foetuses, measure the skull transverse axis, average out the three values and enter them in the formula. **b)** Starting from the foetus transverse axis at the stomach level, obtain the value of the body's transverse diameter. Since the foetus is basically oval, perform two orthogonal measurements and average them out. Repeat it for a minimum of three foetuses. Got this value, enter it into the formula.

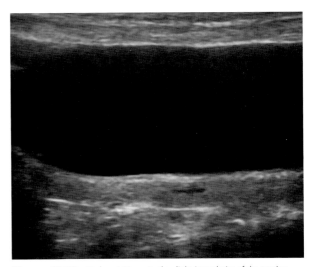

Figure 13.23 Endometritis: note the slight irregularity of the uterine mucous coat and the small accumulation of endoluminal anechoic material.

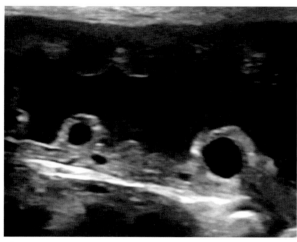

Figure 13.24 Fluid material rich in hyperechoic foci that relaxes the uterine lumen of this patient. The wall is uneven and thickened and contains several huge endometrial cysts. Note the difference between the content of uterine cysts and the uterine contents. These ultrasonographic features are typical of a pyometra, confirmed at surgery. Unfortunately, the appearance of both the endoluminal content and the wall is highly variable and not always differentiable by a hydrometra.

UTERINE STUMP DISEASE (Fig. 13.25)
- Infection of the surgical site the uterine stump was removed from
- Tissues surrounding the stump are hyperechoic and show distal echoes dispersion
- The reactive area may include an anechoic collection, creating the impression of a complex mass.

UTERINE TORSION
- A rare disease, more common in large breed dogs in late pregnancy
- Aspecific ultrasonographic signs, difficult diagnosis
- The most characteristic ultrasonographic sign is a huge asymmetry of uterine horns fluid content: the twisted horn contains much more fluid, rich in hyperechoic foci
- The wall of twisted horn is thickened and hyperechoic

- Foetuses contained in the twisted uterine horn are dead; if diagnosed early, foetuses of the untwisted uterine horn may be alive
- You can hardly observe the twisted wall, but the fluid content in excess is clearly 'saccate' and localized.

ENDOCRINE DISEASES

The most common are uterine cysts, hydrometra and mucometra.

UTERINE CYSTS (Fig. 13.26)
- The endometrial cystic hyperplasia causes an endometrial thickening with formation of anechoic cysts in the thickness of the uterine wall as a result of endometrial glands proliferation
- There is often associated with the build up of endoluminal fluid that predisposes to the formation of hydrometra, mucometra or pyometra.

HYDROMETRA (Fig. 13.27)
- A build up of endoluminal fluid secreted by endometrial glands, sterile and poor in mucin, so anechoic
- The fluid is anechoic and lacks of echoic foci
- The wall is thin and smooth. It can evolve into a pyometra: the two disease are not differentiable by only ultrasonography
- Any significant anechoic uterine collection must always raise a suspicion of pyometra, although it could be a hydrometra.

MUCOMETRA (Fig. 13.28)
- A build up of endoluminal fluid secreted by endometrial glands, sterile and rich in mucin (Fig. 13.28a)
- The endoluminal material is compact and evenly echoic
- It can become infected and turn into a pyometra; in early stages a less echoic area is identifiable within the echoic material (Fig. 13.28b).

UTERINE NEOPLASTIC DISEASES (Fig. 13.29)
Uterine neoplasms are rare in dogs and cats, but the most common are adenomas, adenocarcinomas, leiomyomas and leiomyosarcomas

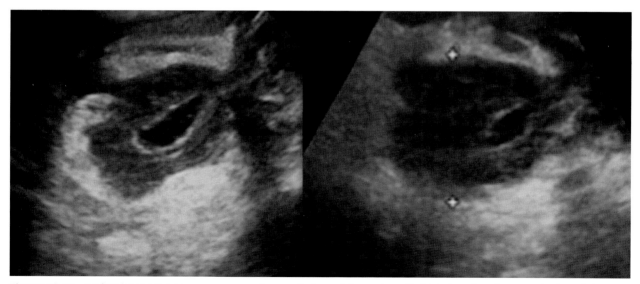

Figure 13.25 A infected uterine stump can appear as a complex mass: the hyperechoic mesentery with distal echoes dispersion surrounds a hypoechoic formation containing a cavity with anechoic material.

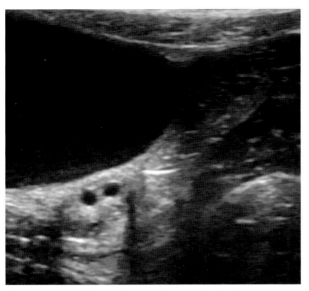

Figure 13.26 Endometrial cysts in the uterus of a female cat.

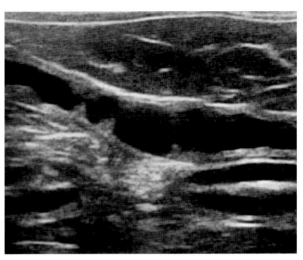

Figure 13.27 Endoluminal collection of anechoic material not associated with a thickening of the uterine wall. In this case it was a hydrometra, but you cannot differentiate it from a pyometra by solely diagnostic imaging. The hydrometra is a predisposing factor for the development of a pyometra.

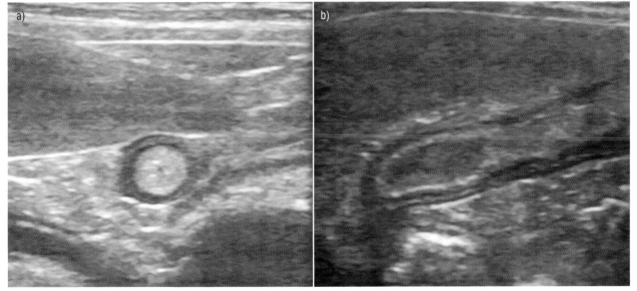

Figure 13.28 **a)** The uterine lumen contains a uniformly echoic material. This finding is typical of mucometra. **b)** Part of the uterus shows a small collection of less echoic material: most likely, this mucometra is becoming a pyometra.

- They appear as nodules or masses, with various shapes, sizes and echostructure
- They can be associated with a build up of endoluminal fluid
- Leiomyomas tend to be isoechoic compared to surrounding uterine tissues, although they may undergo cystic degeneration (Fig. 13.29).

OVARIAN DISEASES

The most common ovarian diseases of ultrasonographic interest are endocrine diseases and neoplastic diseases.

OVARIAN CYSTS (Fig. 13.30)
- Cysts are the most common endocrine ovarian disease

- They appear as well-defined structures, with thin wall and anechoic content, larger than follicular structures. The literature reported that ovarian cysts must exceed 2 cm in diameter; however you can have also hormone-secreting structures with lower diameters
- Distally, there is a posterior-wall enhancement
- They can be single or multiple
- They may be hormone-secreting or non-functional.

OVARIAN NEOPLASMS (Fig. 13.31)
- They are rare in dogs, very rare in cats
- There are four classes of neoplasms:
  - Neoplasms of epithelial origin (40%)
  - Gonadal stromal (50%)
  - Germ cell neoplasms (about 10%)
  - Mesenchymal primary neoplasms (very rare)

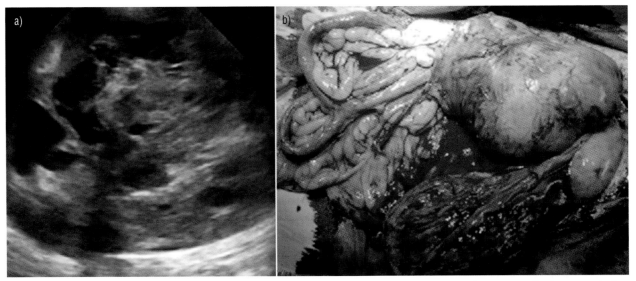

Figure 13.29   a) Partly cavitary appearance of a uterine body leiomyoma. Although the macroscopic and ultrasonographic appearance **b)**, the tumour is benign and the ovariohysterectomy is decisive.

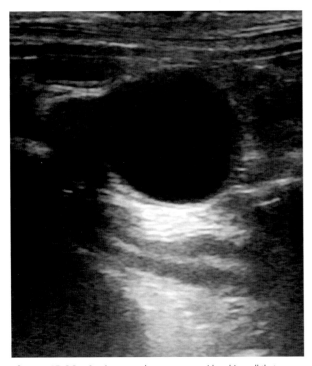

Figure 13.30   Ovarian cyst: a large structure with a thin wall that contains anechoic material and creates a strong posterior-wall enhancement artefact. Sometimes the cyst is so large it makes the ovarian parenchyma identification difficult; in this patient the cyst appears as a hypoechoic oval structure whose cyst changes the caudal pole.

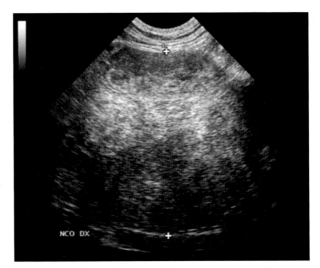

Figure 13.31   Parenchymatous and compact ovarian mass, often diagnosed when a considerable size is reached. They can acquire a cystic appearance.

RECOMMENDED READING

Beccaglia M, Faustini M, Luvoni GC: Ultrasonographic study of deep portion of diencephalo_telencephalic vesicle for the determination of gestational age of the canine foetus. Reprod Dom Anim. 2008, 43: 367–370.

Smith FO: Challenges in small animal parturition—Timing elective and emergency cesarian sections. Theriogenology. 2007, 68: 348–353.

Bang-Sil K, Chang-Ho S: Time of initial detection of foetal and extrafoetal structures by ultrasonographic examination in Miniature Schnauzer Bitches. J. Vet. Sci. 2007, 8(3): 289–293.

Luvoni GC, Beccaglia M: The Prediction of Parturition Date in Canine Pregnancy. Reprod Dom Anim. 2006, 1: 27–32.

Zambelli D, Prati F: Ultrasonography for pregnancy diagnosis and evaluation in queens. Theriogenology. 2006, 66: 135–144.

Kutzler MA, Yeager AE, Mohammed HO, Meyers-Wallen VN: Accuracy of canine parturition date prediction using foetal measurements obtained by ultrasonography. Theriogenology. 2003, 60: 1309–1317.

- On ultrasonography you cannot distinguish which class the neoplasm belongs to. Generally they grow quite large and may appear as:
  - Cystic neoplasms
  - Parenchymal and solid neoplasms (Fig. 13.31)
  - Neoplasms with extensive mineralizations.

Male reproductive system (prostate and testicles)

Luca Benvenuti

SCAN TECHNOLOGY (Fig. 14.1 and 14.2

Animal preparation	• 12 hours on an empty stomach, at least. • Wide hair-clipping. • Good bladder repletion (very important to maintain the prostate in a more cranial position so it can be more easily explored with a transabdominal approach). • Sedation for restless animals, or to make a transrectal examination. • Right and/or left lateral dorsal recumbency. • With patients where the prostate is located very caudally in the pelvis, transabdominal ultrasonography is easier if the body is gently moved cranially using a transrectal acupressure.
Probes	• Microconvex, 7.5 MHz mean frequency (5–10 MHz) for the prostate examination. • Linear, high frequency (7.5–12 MHz), for small breed animals, organ superficial areas and testicles examination.
Prostate: scans and relative position of the probe 	**Transabdominal approach:** • **Longitudinal scan (position 1, Fig. 14.1a and 14.1b):** starting from the bladder longitudinal scan, move the probe caudally towards the bladder trigone to reach the cranial edge of the pubis (Fig. 14.1a). To view the caudal part of the prostatic parenchyma, tilt the probe in the dorsocaudal direction (Fig. 14.1b). From the median position, move right and left to explore the two lobes. • **Transverse scan (position 1, Fig. 14.1c and 14.1d):** starting from the longitudinal scan, rotate the probe by 90° and explore the prostate from the cranial edge to the caudal one (Fig. 14.1c). To view the caudal part of the prostatic parenchyma, tilt the probe in the dorsocaudal direction (Fig. 14.1d). • **Perianal approach (Fig. 14.1e):** very useful with the perianal hernia because the prostate is localized caudally and difficult to see with the transabdominal approach. As an acoustic window you can use the perianal tissues or the anal sphincter. **Transrectal approach:** only possible in medium and large breed dogs, it requires a dedicated probe. Other limits are that you must prepare (enema) and sedate the patient.
Testicles: scans and relative position of the probe	• **Longitudinal scan (Fig. 14.2a):** place the probe directly on the scrotal skin and align it with the testicle longitudinal axis. • **Transverse scan (Fig. 14.2b):** place the probe directly on the scrotal skin, align it with the testicle transverse axis and explore the organ from the cranial edge to the caudal one. If you do not have a high-frequency linear probe, a spacer is needed; alternatively you can use the contralateral testicle as a spacer.

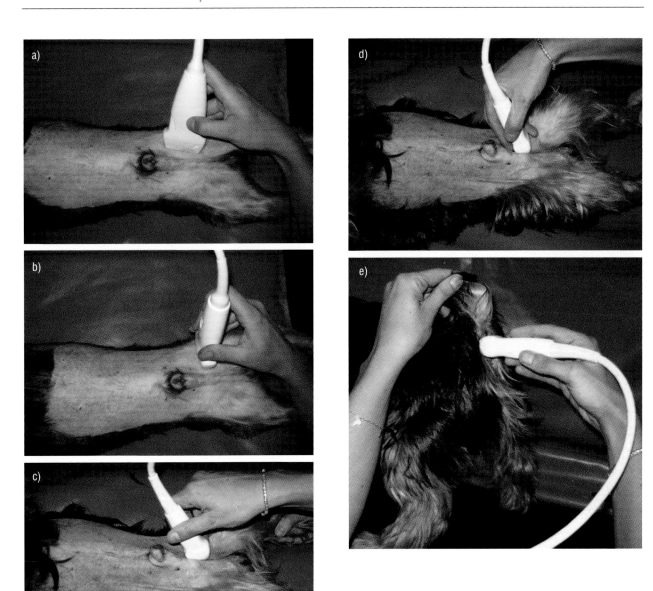

Figure 14.1 Positions for the longitudinal scan **a)** and the transverse scan **c)** of the prostate. To explore the intrapelvic caudal portion of the organ you must tilt the probe in the dorsocaudal direction **(b and d)**. **e)** Perianal approach.

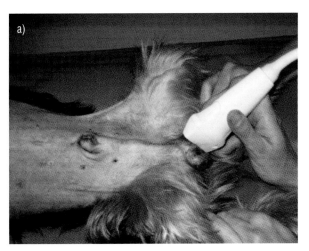
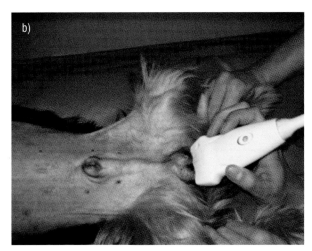

Figure 14.2 Positions for the longitudinal scan **a)** and the transverse scan **c)** of the testicle.

ULTRASONOGRAPHIC ANATOMY (Fig. 14.3–6)

Location	• **Prostate:** caudal abdomen and cranial part of the pelvis, it surrounds the proximal part of the urethra. • **Testicles:** ventral perineal region in dogs and subanal area in cats.
Prostatic morphology	• **Longitudinal scan (Fig. 14.3a):** rounded/oval shape, made from a homogeneous parenchyma and surrounded by a hyperechoic capsule. The urethra appears as a hypoechoic and linear structure that subdivides a dorsal part and a ventral one. • **Transverse scan (Fig. 14.3b):** spherical shape and subdivided into two symmetrical lobes. The urethra is centrally visible, slightly shifted dorsally, hypoechoic; it becomes more visible and shows a higher diameter at the seminal colliculus where the vasa deferentia merge (caudal half of the organ). This hypoechoic area should not be confused with a prostatic injury. The prostate is surrounded by a hyperechoic capsule that is visible when the ultrasound beam is exactly perpendicular to the capsule.
Testicular morphology	• **Longitudinal scan (Fig. 14.4a):** oval, externally delimited by the hyperechoic tunica albuginea. In the middle you see a hyperechoic line that crosses it longitudinally (mediastinum testis). • **Transverse scan (Fig. 14.4b):** round shape, delimited by the hyperechoic tunica albuginea; a hyperechoic dot-like structure in the centre (mediastinum testis). • **Epididymis (Fig. 14.4c):** hypoechoic or anechoic structure located dorsomedially to the testicular parenchyma; it includes a head, a body and a tail (adjacent to the caudal pole).
Prostate: relationships with adjacent organs evaluable on ultrasonography	• **ranially:** bladder neck, perivesical mesenteric tissue. • **Ventrally:** pubis. • **Dorsolaterally:** descending colon and rectum; often, the descending colon is shifted slightly to the left of the midline; going caudally in the pubis, the rectum takes a more dorsal and median position. • **Dorsally:** sublumbar muscles, lumbosacral vertebrae. • **Centrally:** prostatic urethra, which runs longitudinally within the prostatic parenchyma.
Prostate sizes (Table 14.1)	• **Dog:** variable sizes according to the breed size and the patient age (see Table 14.1). The author's clinical experience, supported by unpublished empirical data (average of a thousand not-neutered male dogs aged three to five years, Utrecht University), allows you to relate the dog weight with the normal diameter of the prostate as follows: − <10 kg: 3 cm − <25 kg: 4 cm − >25 kg: 5 cm • **Neutered dog:** small and hypoechoic due to atrophy (Fig. 14.5). If the dog is neutered at a young age, the prostate tends to be homogeneous; if the patient is neutered due to prostatic diseases, we might have an irregular parenchyma. • **Cat:** difficult to examine, being hypoechoic and small sized; the prostate becomes visible in adult not-neutered animals, while it is rarely possible to identify in neutered cats
Testicles sizes	• Variable sizes according to patient size, weight and age. • Undescended testicles are often atrophic, but the atrophy can also be caused by a sertolioma of the contralateral testicle (feminization syndrome, secondary to hyperestrogenism) (Fig. 14.6).
Edges	• Smooth and regular.
Echogenicity	• **Prostate:** slightly more echoic compared to the spleen. • **Testicles:** echoic on average.
Echostructure	• **Prostate:** homogeneous and coarse ultrasound texture. • **Testicles:** homogeneous and slightly granular ultrasound texture.
Vessels	• **Prostatic arteries and veins:** they reach the body of the prostate laterally, branching on its surface.
Tributary lymph nodes	**Medial iliac.**

TABLE 14.1 Prostate sizes in not-neutered adult dogs according to the patient age and body weight (Ruel et al. 1998, Atalan et al. 1999)

	Ruel	Atalan
Length (cm)	1.7–6.9	1.8–5.0
Height (transverse scan) (cm)	1.3–4.7	1.4–3.6
Width (cm)	1.8–6.9	1.4–4.3
Volume (cm³)	2.3–80.0	8.1–28.2

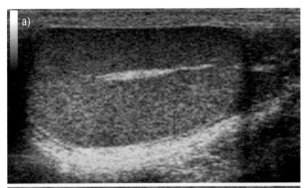

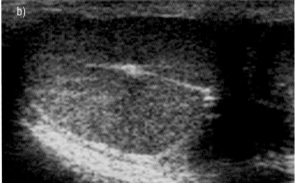

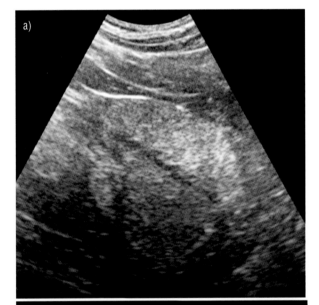

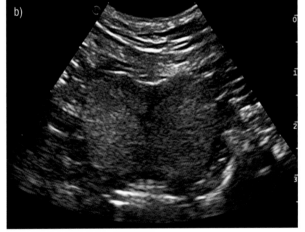

Figure 14.3 Longitudinal scan **a)** and transverse scan **b)** of a normal prostate gland in a not-neutered dog.

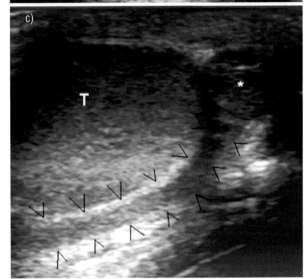

Figure 14.4 Longitudinal scan **a)** and transverse scan **b)** of a normal testicle. **c)** The scan is focused on the epididymis, showing its tail (*) and body (arrowheads).

ULTRASONOGRAPHIC CHANGES

Diffuse parenchymal	• **Prostate:** acute and chronic inflammatory changes, atrophy, metaplasia, neoplasm. • **Testicles:** acute and chronic inflammatory changes, atrophy, torsion, neoplasm.
Focal parenchymal	• **Prostate:** acute and chronic inflammatory changes, cysts, abscesses/granulomas, haematoma, neoplasm. • **Testicles:** neoplasm, cysts, abscesses/granulomas, haematoma.

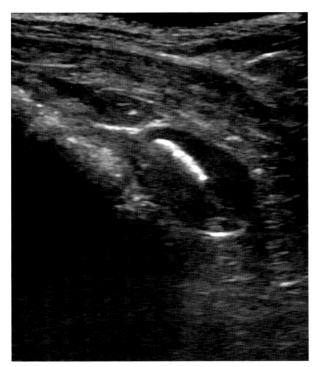

Figure 14.5   Prostatic hypoplasia in a neutered dog: the prostate is small, hypoechoic and homogeneous. Over the prostatic urethra you see a small amount of hyperechoic sediment.

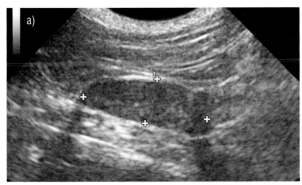

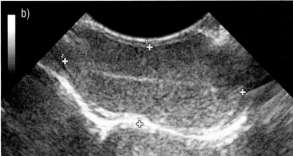

Figure 14.6   a) Undescended testicle, small and hypoechoic (atrophic), in the inguinal position. **b)** Normal contralateral testicle.

PROSTATIC DISEASES

For a proper evaluation of the prostate consider the following ultrasound criteria:

- Geometric abnormalities (size, shape, position and edges). The increase in the prostate size is common with diseases such as benign hyperplasia, prostatitis, or neoplasm
- Parenchymal abnormalities: diffuse or focal changes in echogenicity and echostructure
- Periparenchymal abnormalities: changes in periprostatic fat or adjacent peritoneum with or without effusion.

BENIGN PROSTATIC HYPERPLASIA, CYSTIC PROSTATIC HYPERPLASIA AND PROSTATIC METAPLASIA (Fig. 14.7 and 14.8)

The prostatic hyperplasia is very common in adult dogs (already reported at two years of age), and it is reported in 100 per cent of subjects over seven years.

It is frequently associated with parenchymal cysts, easily subject to infection.

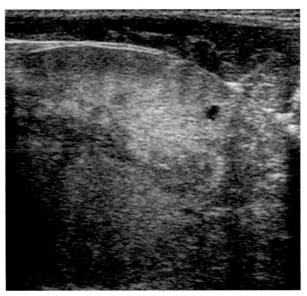

Figure 14.7   Benign prostatic hyperplasia. The prostate is larger and shows irregularly shape and heterogeneous hyperechoic parenchyma with a small parenchymal cyst.

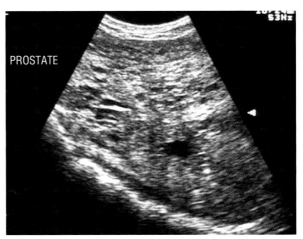

Figure 14.8   Squamous metaplasia in a dog. The longitudinal scan of the prostate shows a hypoechoic parenchyma and a number of small parenchymal cysts.

The prolonged administration or the oestrogen production by some testicular tumours (sertolioma) may cause a squamous metaplasia of the prostate, with tendency to stasis and consequent formation of cysts.

Ultrasonographic findings include:

- Mild/moderate enlargement
- Symmetrical shape if there are no peripheral cysts, at least
- Smooth and regular edges
- Usually higher parenchyma echogenicity, in a homogeneous or heterogeneous way
- Single or multiple anechoic injuries (cysts), usually <1.5 cm
- Normal iliac lymph nodes
- Normal adjacent peritoneum.

BACTERIAL PROSTATITIS (Fig. 14.9–12)
The ultrasonographic appearance features:

- Increased volume
- Changed echogenicity, which varies from diffusely hypoechoic to heterogeneous hyperechoic caused by areas of haemorrhage, fibrosis or mineralization (in chronic forms)
- Hypoechoic-anechoic formations, due to abscessual injuries, areas of oedema, haemorrhage or parenchyma necrosis. Gas accumulations are visible within abscessual formations
- Medial iliac lymphadenomegaly
- Possible changes of periprostatic tissues (effusion, thickening and hyperechogenicity of adjacent tissues, caused by peritonitis and steatitis).

The ultrasonographic differentiation between cystic hyperplasia and prostatitis with abscesses may be difficult based on the sole ultrasonographic presentation and requires a confirmation

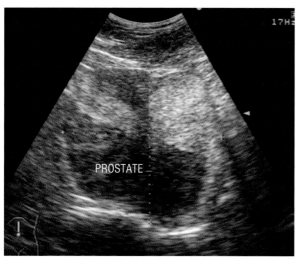

Figure 14.9 Acute prostatitis, transverse scan. The gland is increased in volume, the shape is normal and the parenchyma is heterogeneous with clearly hypoechoic areas compatible with oedema, haemorrhage or necrosis of the parenchyma.

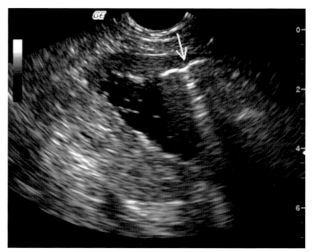

Figure 14.11 Prostatic abscess that is a predominantly anechoic injury containing hyperechoic material. Note the hyperechoic interface (arrow) associated with the characteristic comet tail artefact generated by the small amount of gas within the abscess.

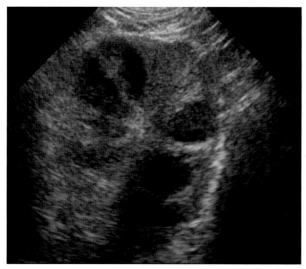

Figure 14.10 Acute prostatitis with multiple abscesses, transverse scan. The prostate is hypoechoic and contains rounded/oval injuries with hypoechoic content. The needle aspiration demonstrated the presence of pus.

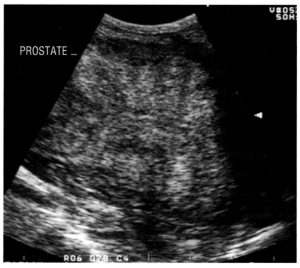

Figure 14.12 Chronic prostatitis. The prostate keeps a normal form, the parenchyma is heterogeneous with striated appearance, caused by organ fibrosis secondary to inflammation. In this case, there are no parenchyma mineralizations.

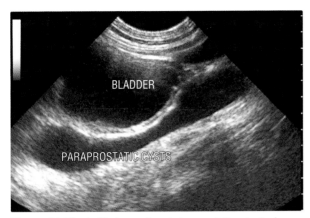

Figure 14.13 In this dog, an elongated paraprostatic cyst extends dorsally to the bladder reaching its cranial edge.

by needle aspiration and subsequent cytological examination and/or the culture.

The iliac lymphadenopathy and changes of the surrounding peritoneum are important diagnostic elements for the differential diagnosis.

PARAPROSTATIC CYSTS (Fig. 14.13)

These cysts extend outside the prostatic parenchyma and are connected to the latter by means of a stalk. The cysts' localization may be abdominal (adjacent to the bladder, lateral or even cranial to it) or in the pelvic canal (adjacent to the rectum, but they may extend caudally to the perineal region; in this case, they are easy to visualize through a perianal approach).

Ultrasonographic findings:

- Anechoic roundish formations separated by a thin wall. Sometimes, the content becomes rich of echoic foci or material (due to haemorrhage or cell collections)
- Variable sizes (up to tens of cm in diameter)
- Sometimes subdivided by hyperechoic septa
- Often associated with a prostatic disease (benign hyperplasia or prostatitis).

If the paraprostatic cyst size is similar to the bladder, it can be difficult to readily differentiate the two structures. To do so, it is important to study its caudal portion, which has a different ending: the bladder continues with the urethra, while the cyst connects with the prostatic parenchyma, although it is not always easy to visualize clearly the stalk that joins them.

NEOPLASM (Fig. 14.14 and 14.15)

Prostatic tumours in dogs are less common than other previously covered prostatic diseases. In dogs the diagnosis is often late (unlike in humans), when the tumour sizes are already considerable. The presence of prostatomegaly and ultrasonographic changes in a neutered dog must raise a strong suspicion of neoplasm.

Ultrasonographic findings include:

- Increased volume
- Often asymmetrical shape
- The capsule may appear normal, irregular or show irregularities caused by the invasion of surrounding tissues

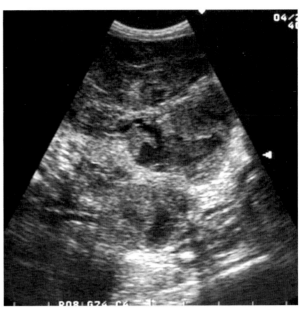

Figure 14.14 Prostatic adenocarcinoma. The prostate is enlarged, with very irregular shape and capsule irregularities. The parenchyma is heterogeneous with anechoic and hypoechoic areas.

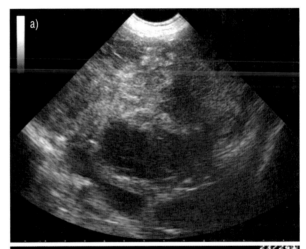

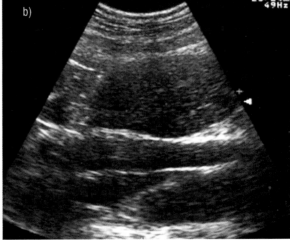

Figure 14.15 Another example of prostatic carcinoma, where the prostate contains bulky hypoechoic cavities caused by necrosis and/or haemorrhages **a)** The medial iliac lymph node of the same dog **b)** is enlarged and hypoechoic, due to its metastatic involvement.

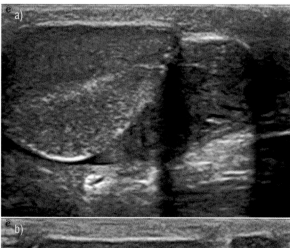

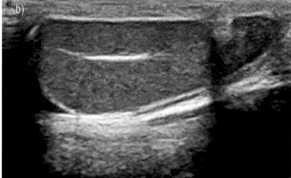

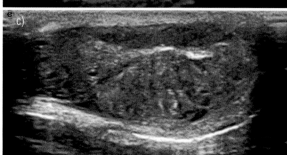

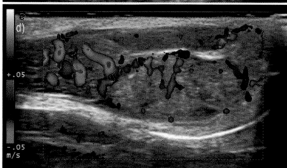

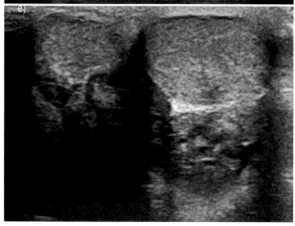

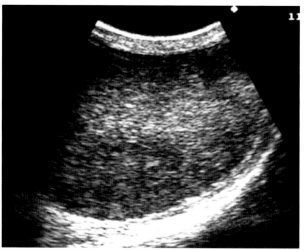

Figure 14.17 Chronic orchitis. The testicle appears markedly hyperechoic and heterogeneous.

- Diffusely heterogeneous parenchyma
- Dot-like hyperechoic mineralizations. Although mineralizations may be associated to chronic prostatitis, their frequency is higher in neoplasms
- Cavitary injuries with necrotic or cystic origin
- Lymphadenopathy of medial iliac lymph nodes or hypogastric or sacral lymph nodes
- Other metastatic injuries. The most metastasised organs, beyond regional lymph nodes, are pelvis, lumbar vertebrae, peritoneum and lungs. The radiographic examination is mandatory to evaluate skeletal structures and lungs.

TESTICULAR DISEASES

ORCHITIS (Fig. 14.16 and 14.17)

The inflammatory testicular pictures are often associated with epididymitis.

They are usually secondary to inflammation of the prostate, the bladder and the urethra, or traumas and penetrating foreign bodies. On ultrasonography, they appear as:

- Acute forms: enlarged, with heterogeneous appearance of the parenchyma due to diffuse injuries (hypoechoic dot-like). You may also view hypoechoic or anechoic abscessual injuries with irregular edges
- Chronic forms: heterogeneous appearance of the parenchyma with hyperechoic areas caused by fibrosis. Reduced sizes due to the contributory atrophy.

Sometimes it is difficult to differentiate an acute inflammatory picture from a neoplastic one; this is only possible through a cytological or histopathological examination.

◀ **Figure 14.16** Acute unilateral orchitis-epididymitis. **a)** The testicle and the epididymis are enlarged. This is clear when compared to the normal contralateral testicle **b)**; the epididymis is heterogeneous **c)** and shows a marked vascularization **d)**. **e)** Transverse scan of both testicles and epididymides.

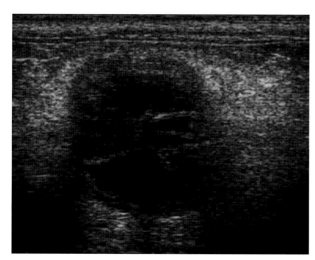

Figure 14.18 Torsion of an undescended testicle in the abdominal position. The testicle appears markedly hypoechoic compared to the surrounding peritoneum, and slightly heterogeneous. The adjacent peritoneum is thickened and hyperechoic. The Colour Doppler study (not shown) did not show any evidence of parenchymal flow.

TORSION (Fig. 14.18)

It can occur in both undescended testicles and scrotal testicles. Ultrasonographic changes are visible quickly, from 15 to 60 minutes after the torsion.

It should be noted:

- Enlargement
- Diffuse hypoechogenicity of the parenchyma
- Reduction of vascularization seen at Colour Doppler
- Changes of the adjacent peritoneum associated to undescended testicle (effusion or signs of peritonitis).

NEOPLASMS (Fig. 14.19 and 14.20)

Testicular neoplasms include interstitial cell tumours (leydigomas or interstiziomas), sertoliomas and seminomas. In cryptorchids the incidence of testicular neoplasms increases, and these tumours have a more aggressive biological behaviour than tumours of scrotal testicles, with higher frequency of metastases in lymph nodes and other organs.

Ultrasonographic findings:

- Neoplasms usually appear as single or multiple nodules located within a normal or enlarged testicle
- There are no particular ultrasonographic features to differentiate the different neoplastic pictures; the appearance may be homogeneous (hyperechoic or hypoechoic) or heterogeneous with anechoic areas referable to cysts, haemorrhage or necrosis
- With tumours producing feminizing hormones (sertolioma), the contralateral testicle may appear atrophic
- The evaluation of medial iliac lymph nodes is paramount to searching for any regional metastases.

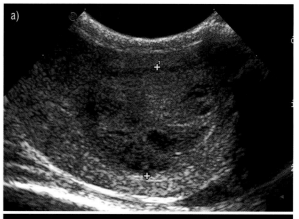
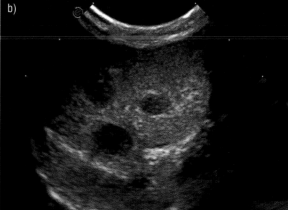
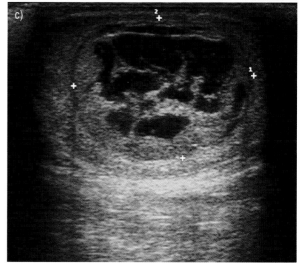

Figure 14.20 Examples of testicular neoplasms, in the form of testicular nodules with a heterogeneous **a)**, hypoechoic **b)** or cystic **c)** appearance.

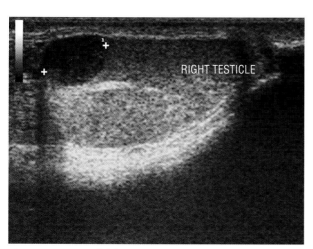

Figure 14.19 Well-defined hypoechoic testicular nodule (final diagnosis, leydigoma).

RECOMMENDED READING

Atalan G, Holt PE, Barr FJ. Ultrasonographic estimation of prostate size in normal dogs and relationship to bodyweight and age. J Small Anim Pract 1999; 40: 119–122.

Johnston GR, Feeney DA, Rivers B, Walter PA. Diagnostic imaging of the male canine reproductive organs: Methods and limitations. Vet Clin North Am Small Anim Pract 1991; 21: 553–559.

Robert E. Cartee and Terri Rowles. Transabdominal sonographic evaluation of the canine prostate. Veterinary radiology 1983; 24: 156–164.

Kaitkanoke Kamolpatana, Gary R Johnston and Shirley D Johnston. Determination of canine prostatic volume using transabdominal ultrasonography. Veterinary radiology & ultrasound 2000; 41: 73–77.

Gultekin Atalan, Frances J Barr and Peter E Holt. Comparison of ultrasonographic and radiographic measurements of canine prostate dimensions. Veterinary radiology & ultrasound 1999; 40: 408–412.

Jonathan L Stowater and Christopher R Lamb. Ultrasonographic features of paraprostatic cysts in nine dogs. Veterinary radiology 1989; 30: 232–239.

Bradbury CA, Westropp JI and Pollard RE. Relationship between prostatomegaly, prostatic mineralization, and cytologic diagnosis. Veterinary radiology & ultrasound 2009; 50: 167–171.

15 Upper urinary tract (kidney and ureter)

Luca Benvenuti

SCAN TECHNOLOGY (Fig. 15.1A, B)

Animal preparation	• 12 hours on an empty stomach, at least. • Wide hair-clipping, including intercostal spaces. • Sedation for restless animals or to perform biopsies. • Right and/or left lateral dorsal recumbency.
Probes	• Microconvex, 7.5 MHz mean frequency (5–10 MHz). • Linear, high frequency (7.5–12 MHz), for small breed animals and organs' superficial portions.
Scans and respective probe position – left kidney 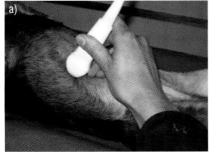	• Sagittal longitudinal scan, median (position 4) and dorsal (coronal): longitudinally oriented beam with the probe over the middle abdominal region, caudally to the costal arch, ventrally to the lumbar vertebrae L1 to L3. The ultrasound beam crosses the porta renis (dorsal scan) or moves tangentially to it (sagittal scan). Approaching the kidney ventrally with the animal in dorsal recumbency, a certain pressure is often necessary to move the colon laterally or medially. If the animal is in the lateral recumbency, the needed pressure is lower and the kidney tends to move more towards the centre of the abdomen. Rarely, if the left kidney position is very cranial, an intercostal approach from the last intercostal space is used. • Transverse scan: transversely oriented beam with the probe over the dorsal abdominal region of the left flank, caudally to the costal arch and ventrally to lumbar vertebrae L1 to L3 (starting from position 4, rotation by 90 degrees).
Scans and respective probe position – right kidney	• Longitudinal scans: median sagittal (position 9, Fig. 15.1a) and dorsal (coronal, Fig. 15.1b); longitudinally oriented beam with the probe over the abdominal middle region, just caudally to the costal arch. The ultrasound beam crosses the porta renis (dorsal scan) or moves tangentially to it (sagittal scan). The ventral approach is more difficult and requires some pressure, especially in large breed animals as various organs interpose between the skin and the kidney (ascending colon, pylorus, and duodenum). If unsatisfactory, the intercostal approach is used. • Transverse scan (Fig. 15.1c): transversely oriented beam with the probe over the dorsal abdominal region of the right flank, caudally to the hypochondrium or between last two intercostal spaces (starting from position 4, rotation by 90 degrees). • Intercostal scans: the probe over last two intercostal spaces, caudally to the caudate liver lobe.

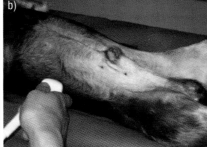

Figure 15.1 Probe positions for longitudinal sagittal median **(a)**, dorsal or coronal **(b)**, and transverse **(c)** scans.

ULTRASONOGRAPHIC ANATOMY (Fig. 15.2, 15.3, 15.4 and 15.5, Diagrams 15.1 and 15.2)

Location	• Cranial lumbar region of the left and right flank.
Morphology	• Shape: oval (sagittal scan) or bean-shaped (dorsal scan crossing the hilum). • Capsule: thin hyperechoic interface, clearly visible where the ultrasound beam strikes it at right angles. • Cortex: peripheral; similar thickness to the medullary. • Medullary: internal; lobules subdivided by hyperechoic lines representing the walls of interlobar vessels and the renal diverticula. The medullary thickness is similar to the cortex. • Renal crest: an extension of the medullary that separates it from the pelvis; hyperechoic. • Pelvis: located in the centre of a hyperechoic area (sinus) and made of adipose tissue; the pelvis lumen is visible especially if slightly dilated (animal that is polyuric, under infusion, or treated with diuretics).
Right kidney: relationships with adjacent organs evaluable on ultrasonography	• Cranially: caudate process of the caudate liver lobe. • Caudally: right ovary and jejunal loops. • Ventrally: descending duodenum, right pancreatic lobe, ascending colon, caudal vena cava and right adrenal gland (medially). • Dorsally: lumbar vertebrae.
Left kidney: relationships with adjacent organs evaluable on ultrasonography	• Cranially: greater curvature of the stomach, spleen, left pancreatic lobe. • Caudally: left ovary, jejunal loops and descending colon. • Ventrally: spleen, jejunal loops, descending colon. • Dorsally: left adrenal gland (medially) and aorta.
Size	• Dog: variable size in relation to the patient breed size. Mareschal et al. proposed a method to evaluate renal size (adult animal) by calculating the ratio between the kidney length (L) and the aorta diameter (Ao), measured at the porta renis. The L/Ao ratio must be between 5.5 and 9.1. • Cat: the bibliography reports following values:

Feline kidney size (cm)	Walter et al., 1987	Nickel et al., 1973
Length	3.66 ±0.46	3.8–4.4
Thickness	2.53 ±0.30	2.7–3.1
Height	2.21 ±0.28	2.0–2.5

• Medullary and pelvis may enlarge in animals with increased diuresis (PU-PD, infusion, diuretics treatment). |
Edges	• Smooth and regular.
Echogenicity relationship (Fig. 15.4 and 15.5)	• Dog: renal medullary < renal cortex < liver < spleen. • Cat: renal medullary < renal cortex (common cortex hyperechogenicity compared to the liver parenchyma due to physiological infiltration of fat vacuoles).
Echostructure	• Fine and homogeneous cortex echostructure. • Distinct boundary between cortex and medullary (corticomedullary junction).
Vessels	• Renal arteries and veins: visible over the hilum and distinguishable by using the Doppler feature. • Arcuate arteries: visible at the corticomedullary junction; walls form pairs of interfaces that can produce shadowing and should not be confused with areas of mineralization. • Interlobar arteries: distinguishable in the medullary by oblique scans and the Doppler feature.
Tributary lymph nodes	• Renal.

Diagram 15.1

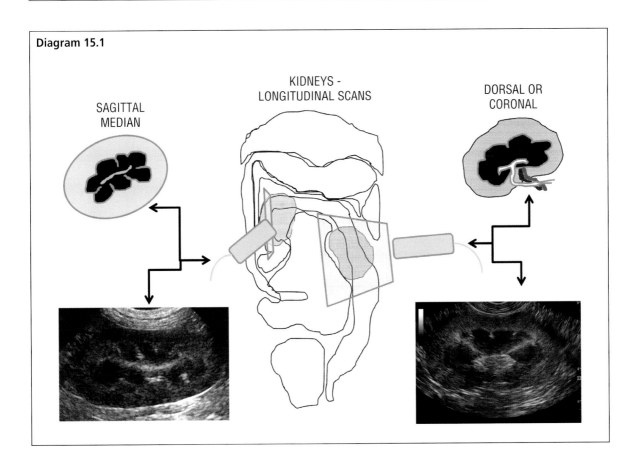

Diagram 15.2

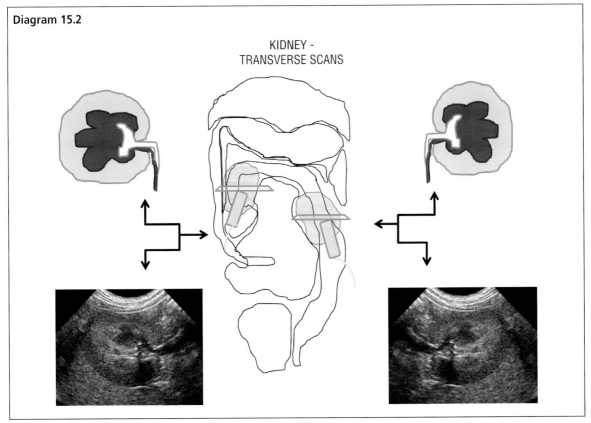

Diagrams 15.1 and 15.2 show scans investigating kidneys and related ultrasonographic images in dogs.

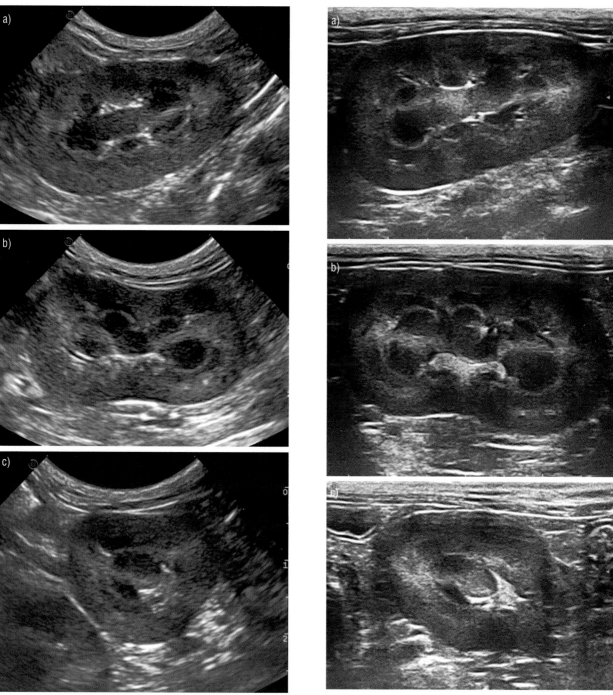

Figure 15.2 Ultrasonographic images of a feline kidney, micro-convex probe. Sagittal longitudinal, median **(a)**, dorsal **(b)** and transverse **(c)** scans.

Figure 15.3 Ultrasonographic images of a feline kidney, linear probe. Sagittal longitudinal, median **(a)**, dorsal **(b)** and transverse **(c)** scans.

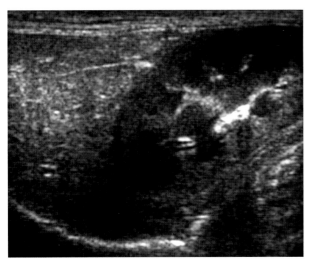

Figure 15.4   Kidney/liver echogenicity ratio in dogs.

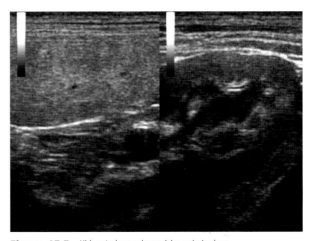

Figure 15.5   Kidney/spleen echogenicity ratio in dogs.

ULTRASONOGRAPHIC CHANGES - KIDNEY

Diffuse parenchymal	Congenital diseases (familial nephropathies or renal dysplasia) Fig. 15.6 and 15.7. Acquired diseases: • Acute and chronic inflammation (glomerulonephritis, interstitial nephritis). • Nephrosis and tubular necrosis. • Nephrocalcinosis. • Primary neoplasm (e.g. lymphoma).
Focal parenchymal	• Cysts. • Abscesses. • Haematoma. • Infarctions. • Stones. • Primary or secondary neoplasm (metastases, often multifocal).
Collector system diseases	• Pyelectasis and hydronephrosis. • Nephrolithiasis. • Pyelonephritis.
Perirenal diseases	• Perirenal pseudocysts (cat). • Inflammations (acute nephritis) and FIP (cat). • Neoplasm (e.g. lymphoma). • Trauma.

CONGENITAL ABNORMALITIES

Familial nephropathies (renal dysplasias) (Fig. 15.6 and 15.7) affect dogs from four months to two–three years. They have been described in 20 breeds at least (Bull Terrier, Chow-Chow, Cocker Spaniel, Dobermann Pinscher, Lhasa Apso, Shih Tzu, Samoyed, Boxer, Poodle, etc.). The disease is caused by a disorganized development of the renal parenchyma and evolves in severe progressive bilateral glomerular, periglomerular or interstitial fibrosis, in glomerular and tubular atrophy, and may be associated to cysts. On ultrasonography, the kidney appears:

• Normal to reduced
• Irregularly shaped
• Diffusely hyperechoic

• With poor corticomedullary appearance
• The pelvis may be normal or enlarged.

DIFFUSE PARENCHYMAL CHANGES

They can be associated with cortex hyperechogenicity or hypoechogenicity. The cortex diffuse hyperechogenicity does not mean a specific nephropathy, but may be seen in case of:

• Acute tubular necrosis
• Early-stage fibrosis
• Nephritis: glomerulonephritis, interstitial nephritis, pyelonephritis (associated with pyelectasis), granulomatous nephritis (FIP)
• Hypercalcaemic nephropathy

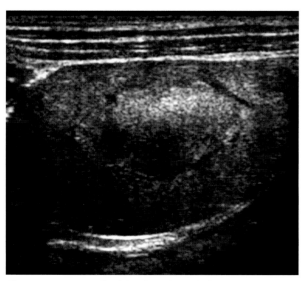

Figure 15.6 Boxer, familial nephropathy. The kidney lost its normal corticomedullary architecture and is diffusely hyperechoic.

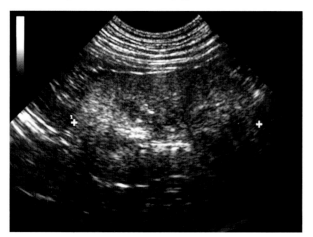

Figure 15.7 Dog, renal dysplasia.

- Ethylene glycol poisoning
- Infiltrative diseases (amyloidosis, lymphoma, squamous cell carcinoma).

The definitive diagnosis can be established with lab tests and renal tissue biopsy.

Depending on the disease stage, ultrasonographic findings vary (Fig. 15.8–12):

- In acute forms (e.g. acute toxic or inflammatory) the kidney shape is preserved, sizes range from normal to slightly enlarged, and the architecture is preserved. The cortex hyperechogenicity enhances the corticomedullary distinction
- With advanced or end-stage chronic renal diseases, the kidney tends to be small (end-stage kidney) and irregularly shaped. The increased echogenicity affects also the medullary, resulting in diffuse hyperechoic appearance of the kidney and poor corticomedullary distinction. Areas of mineralization are common and sometimes difficult to differentiate from kidney stones.

The 'medullary rim sign' (Fig. 15.13) is a medullary hyperechoic band close and parallel to the corticomedullary junction.

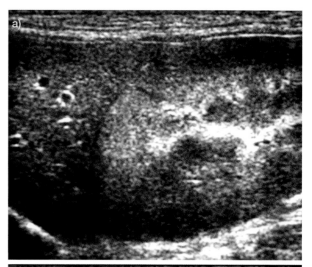

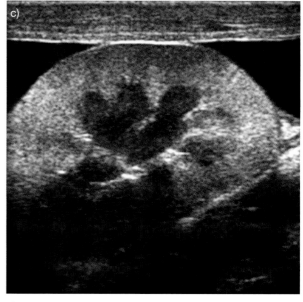

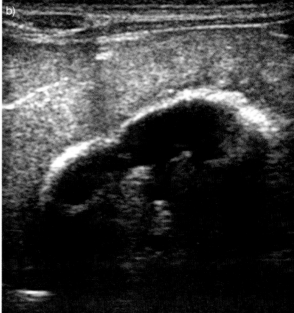

Figure 15.8 Examples of hyperechogenicity and cortex thickening with preserved kidney shape. **a)** Dog with acute glomerulonephritis. **b)** Dog with ethylene glycol poisoning; a clear medullary rim sign is also shown. **c)** Renal amyloidosis in a cat.

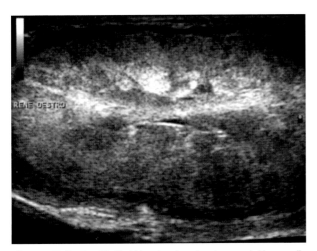

Figure 15.9 Cat, FIP. The kidney is enlarged and surrounded by a small amount of perirenal effusion. The cortex and the medullary are hyperechoic with small hypoechoic nodular injuries. The superficial small granulomas alter the kidney, whose surface appears bumpy.

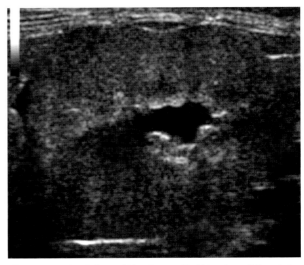

Figure 15.12 End-stage kidney in a cat. The kidney is small, irregularly shaped and lost its normal corticomedullary architecture. The pelvis is slightly enlarged.

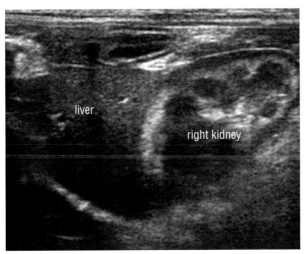

liver

right kidney

Figure 15.10 Dog, interstitial nephritis. The cortex thickness is reduced and the inner portion is decidedly hyperechoic compared to the adjacent liver parenchyma.

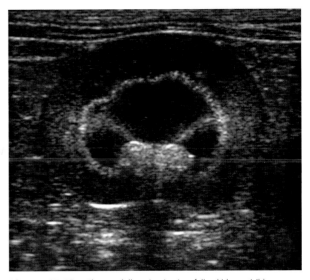

Figure 15.13 Clear medullary rim sign in a feline kidney, visible as hyperechoic medullary band close and parallel to the corticomedullary junction.

The meaning of this ultrasonographic sign is still not fully clarified.

It can be associated with several kidney diseases (hypercalcaemic nephropathy, ethylene glycol poisoning, leptospirosis, renal lymphoma, infectious peritonitis).

Histologically, the injury corresponds to tubular damage with calcification of the basement membrane of the Bowman's capsule and of the tubular epithelium, which occurs in the innermost portion of the medullary.

However, especially in feline species, the 'medullary rim sign' is also visible in clinically normal patients.

Some authors suggest that it may be a preclinical sign of kidney disease, although this theory was not scientifically proofed.

With infiltrative neoplasms and renal vein thrombosis associated with increased parenchymal volume, a cortex hypoechogenicity can be detected (e.g. lymphoma or mast cell tumour) (Fig. 15.14).

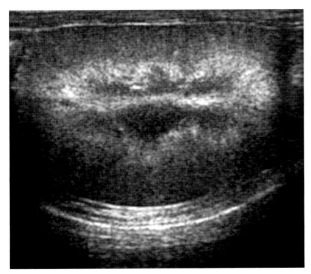

Figure 15.11 Cat, chronic nephritis. The kidney is small, the cortex is hyperechoic and the corticomedullary junction is difficult to define.

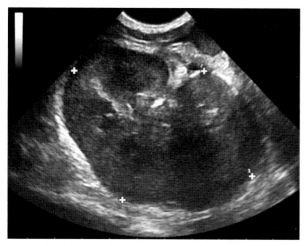

Figure 15.14 Hypoechogenicity and cortex diffuse thickening in a cat with renal lymphoma.

FOCAL PARENCHYMAL CHANGES

They include:

- Cysts
- Abscesses
- Haematoma
- Neoplasms
- Cysts (Fig. 15.15) appear as injuries:
- Rounded or oval
- Associated with posterior-wall enhancement (missing in solid injuries)
- Usually anechoic; if complicated with haemorrhage or infection the content becomes more echoic
- Sometimes subdivided by hyperechoic septa
- In cats suffering from Polycystic Kidney Disease (PKD), an inherited disease common in longhair cats and Persians, cystic injuries sometimes numerous can lead to severe nephromegaly with renal shape deformation and no residual normal parenchyma.

Abscesses (Fig. 15.16) usually appear as:

- Irregular or encapsulated boundaries
- Anechoic/hypoechoic content with corpuscular component

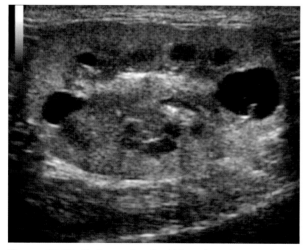

Figure 15.15 Nephromegaly and multiple renal cysts in a cat with PKD.

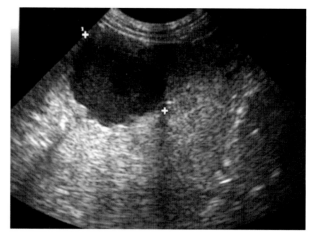

Figure 15.16 Renal abscess with slightly irregular edges and corpuscular hypoechoic content. Note the posterior-wall enhancement, which indicates a fluid content and helps to differentiate the abscess from a hypoechoic solid injury.

- Sometimes there is some gas, visible as a hyperechoic content that produces reverberation artefacts
- Sometimes there are internal mineralizations.

The haematoma has variable size and echogenicity, correlated to the evolutionary stage. Caused by coagulopathies or traumas, haematomas appear as hypoechoic and/or hyperechoic formations with intraparenchymal or subcapsular location; in the latter case, the perirenal pseudocyst must be considered as a differential diagnosis.

Chronic renal infarctions (Fig. 15.17) appear as:

- Triangular hyperechoic injuries with the apex centrally directed and the base directed towards the capsule
- Next to the injury, the renal capsule is usually hollow and the cortex thinned.

Renal neoplasms (Fig. 15.14, 15.18 and 15.19) appear as:

- Focal injuries (primary or metastatic neoplasms)
- Diffuse infiltrative injuries (e.g. lymphoma). The renal lymphoma is associated with nephromegaly, irregular shape

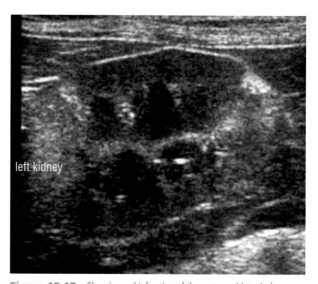

Figure 15.17 Chronic renal infarction of the cortex, with typical hyperechoic and triangular appearance.

and changes in echogenicity that range from diffuse renal hyperechogenicity to a peripheral hypoechoic band of the cortex, and to focal injuries (nodules or masses with variable echogenicity)

- Usually there is a mixed echogenicity due to variable amounts of internal necrosis, fibrosis, haemorrhages, infections and mineralizations. Sometimes, metastases appear as isoechoic nodules within the cortex, so difficult to visualize without a Doppler device or a contrast agent
- With cystadenoma or cystadenocarcinoma (the most common neoplasm in German Shepherd and Golden Retriever, often associated to nodular dermatofibrosis) the cystic component prevails.

Note that ultrasonographic findings described for neoplasms are similar to those of benign injuries. The operator experience is an important factor which often directs towards the correct diagnosis; nevertheless, the benign or malignant nature of the injury is impossible to establish definitively and must be established with a biopsy.

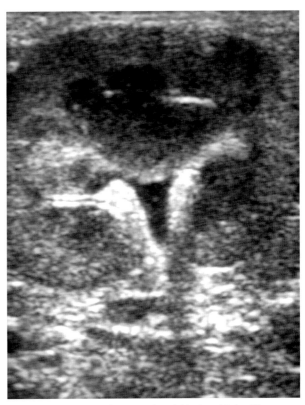

Figure 15.20 Cat with acute pyelonephritis; the pelvis is mildly stretched with a slightly echoic content, while the pelvis wall is hyperechoic.

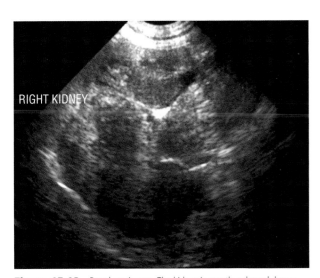

Figure 15.18 Renal carcinoma. The kidney is greatly enlarged, has a rounded shape and has lost its normal architecture. The pelvis position is indicated by the residual hyperechoic peripelvic adipose tissue.

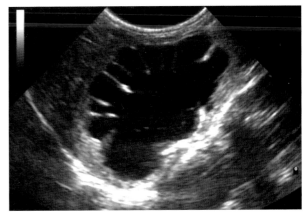

Figure 15.21 Hydronephrosis. The pelvis is greatly expanded with an anechoic content. Thin septa and cortex tissue are visualized, representing the atrophic renal parenchyma.

Collector system diseases include:

- Pyelectasis (Fig. 15.20): early enlargement of the renal pelvis secondary to pyelonephritis, nephrolithiasis or diuretics administration.
- Hydronephrosis (Fig. 15.21): is a more marked dilation of renal pelvis and pelvic diverticula, secondary to ureteral obstruction. As hydronephrosis worsens, the surrounding renal parenchyma undergoes progressive atrophy. In more severe forms, the kidney becomes an anechoic oval structure bounded by a thin capsule, where septa are recognized that correspond to the residual renal parenchyma.
- Nephrolithiasis (Fig. 15.22) With nephrolithiasis, stones appear as hyperechoic formations that produce shadowing,

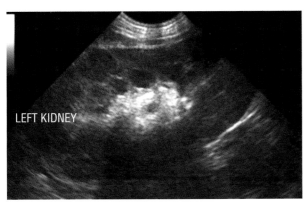

Figure 15.19 Hypoechoic cortex nodule; the cytological examination demonstrated it was a metastasis of a previous thyroid carcinoma.

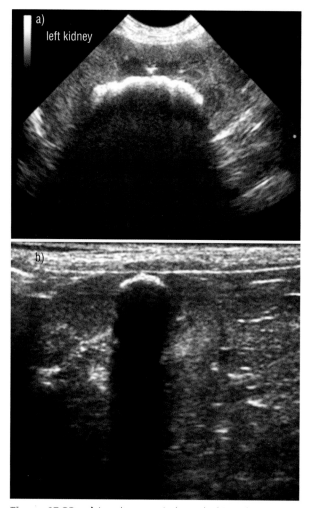

Figure 15.22 a) A staghorn stone in the renal pelvis produces a curvilinear hyperechoic interface with clean shadowing. **b)** Mineralization of the cortex.

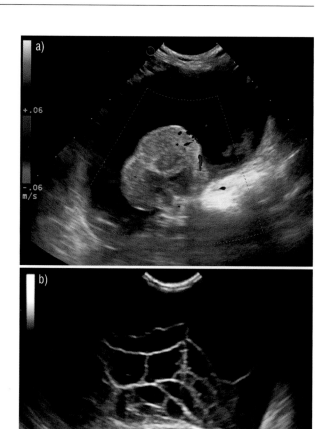

Figure 15.23   Two examples of renal pseudocysts. **a)** Cyst with homogeneous anechoic content; the Doppler shows the residual renal flow. **b)** Pseudocyst with anechoic content subdivided by hyperechoic septa.

located at the diverticula or the pelvis. Small kidney stones are sometimes difficult to differentiate from renal parenchyma mineralizations.

- Pyelitis or acute pyelonephritis (Fig. 15.20): appears as pyelectasis, hyperechogenicity of the pelvis wall and, sometimes, echoic corpuscular material within the pelvis lumen. With pyelonephritis, the kidney may show changes in echogenicity. As the process becomes chronic, a picture of progressive fibrosis arises giving the kidney the appearance of other chronic nephropathies.

PERIRENAL SPACE DISEASES (Fig. 15.23 and 15.24)

The perirenal pseudocysts are perirenal collections bounded by a wall of non-epithelial histological origin.

In cats, they may be secondary to degenerative-inflammatory chronic kidney diseases, FIP, neoplasms or traumas. In these cases, the collection, often in a subcapsular location, surrounds the kidney maintaining an oval shape.

Renal traumas can cause encapsulated collections that appear as pseudocysts (perirenal urinomas). Trauma subjects have not-encapsulated perirenal collections whose shape is more irregular, triangular or linear, as it is distributed in the retroperitoneal space.

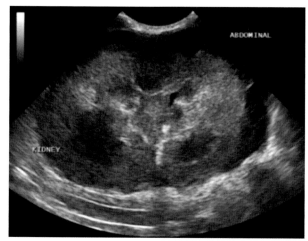

Figure 15.24   Perirenal collection associated to lymphoma in a cat.

The collection can be made by blood, urine or exudate and the ultrasonographic appearance can be similar, even if a higher cellular content (blood or inflammatory cells) increases the echogenicity.

With infections of the retroperitoneal space (secondary to foreign bodies migration, pyelonephritis or urethritis), changes are also observed in the retroperitoneal adipose tissue, which becomes thickened and hyperechoic.

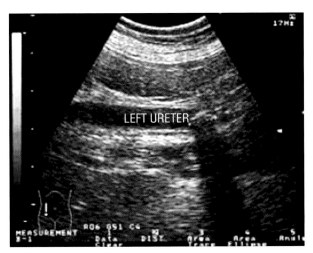

Figure 15.25 Dilation of the proximal portion of a ureter. On the right image a hyperechoic structure is visible that produces shadowing (stone), due to the obstruction.

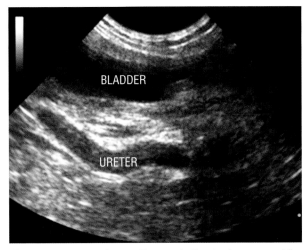

Figure 15.26 Ectopic ureter. The ureter is dilated and goes on caudally beyond its physiological point of termination.

URETER

Normally, the ureter is not visible on ultrasonography unless pathological; this must persuade the ultrasonographer to carefully explore the retroperitoneal space between the kidney and the bladder.

HYDROURETER (Fig. 15.25)

With partial or complete obstruction, the proximal ureteral tract dilates; among leading causes, there are focal inflammations, blood clots, stones or neoplasms of the ureter or the bladder trigone, prolonged bladder or urethral obstructions, compressive retroperitoneal masses, retroperitoneal adhesions or accidental surgical ligatures. Ultrasonographic findings include:

- Tubular structure that can be followed from the renal pelvis caudally in the retroperitoneal space, sometimes up to its termination in the bladder trigone
- Anechoic content (normal urine) or more echoic content (with urinary sediment or urinary tract infection)
- Thin and regular, or more thickened wall in case of inflammation
- The ureter must be followed to search for the possible place and cause of obstruction which can be endoluminal (stone, neoplasm), intramural (wall injury) or extramural (outside compression by cicatricial masses or phenomena).

URETEROCELE

It is a congenital intramural cystic dilation of the ureter, located near the bladder trigone. It appears as a rounded structure associated with the ureterovesical junction, often projecting into the bladder lumen, with an anechoic content. It is often associated with hydroureter, hydronephrosis and urinary tract infection.

PERIURETERAL URINOMA

It is a urine collection externally to the ureter, in the form of a paraureteral pseudocyst, usually secondary to traumatic rupture or intraoperative accidental injury.

URETERAL ECTOPIA (Fig. 15.26)

While not the preferred method to diagnose the ureteral ectopia, the ultrasonography is often helpful when that congenital disease is suspected. As a matter of fact, the ectopic ureter often dilates, so it can be followed in the caudal direction to search for and identify its outlet. If the ureter is ectopic, there is no normal outlet in the trigone and the ureter goes on caudally. Ultrasonographic findings include:

- Dilated ureter
- The ureter does not bend over normally towards the bladder trigone, but goes on in the caudal direction within the pelvis
- Absence of ureteral jet from the ectopic ureter side.

On ultrasonography, stating for certain the outlet location (urethra, vagina) is difficult; therefore, definitive diagnosis has to be determined by descending urography or CT with contrast.

RECOMMENDED READING

Nyland TG, Kantrowitz BM, Fisher P, Olander HJ, Hornof WJ: Ultrasonic determination of kidney volume in the dog. Vet Radiology 1989; 30: 174–180.

Karen L Morrow, Mowafak D. Salman, Michael R. Lappin and Robert Wrigley. Comparison of the resistive index to clinical parameters in dogs with renal disease. Veterinary Radiology & ultrasound 1996; 37: 193–199.

Mantis P and Lamb CR. Most dogs with medullary rim sign on ultrasonography have no demonstrable renal dysfunction. Veterinary radiology & ultrasound 2000; 41: 164–166.

Konde LJ, Wrigley RH, Park RD and Lebel JL. Sonographic appearance of renal neoplasia in the dog. Veterinary radiology 1985; 26: 74–81.

Valdés-martínez, A, Cianciolo R and Mai W. Association between renal hypoechoic subcapsular thickening and lymphosarcoma in cats. Veterinary radiology & ultrasound 2007; 357–360.

Felkai CS, Vörös K, Vrabély T and Karsai F. Ultrasonographic determination of renal volume in the dog. Veterinary radiology & ultrasound 1992; 33: 292–296.

16 Lower urinary tract (bladder and urethra)

Edoardo Auriemma

SCAN TECHNIQUE (Fig. 16.1)

Animal preparation	• Normally repleted bladder. • With hyporepletion, a seemingly thickened wall is visualized (artefact thickening, so the study must be repeated with a normally repleted bladder). • Hair-clipping of the middle-caudal abdomen.
Probes	• Microconvex, 5 MHz mean frequency (3–8 MHz). • Linear, high-frequency (7.5–12 MHz), for small breed animals and organ superficial portions.
Scans and respective probe position	**Bladder** • Transverse scan (position 1): the probe is in contact with the median portion of the caudal abdomen (just cranially to the pubis) and the beam is transversely oriented. From the pubis, the probe is moved cranially, remaining on the median line, perpendicular to the spine, until the bladder is identified (Fig. 16.1a). The organ is explored from the more caudal part to the more cranial portion. • Longitudinal scan (position 1): the probe is in contact with the median portion of the caudal abdomen. After having identified the bladder in cross section, rotate the probe by 90 degrees and obtain a longitudinal scan of the organ (Fig. 16.1b). The organ is explored from left to right. • Oblique scans (position 1): the probe is moved along position 1 to optimize the visualization of bladder portions not completely explorable by the other scans (e.g. bladder neck). **Urethra** • The proximal tract comes up from the bladder neck and goes on caudally to the pubis that creates a clean posterior shadowing preventing its visualization. The female urethra, when normal, is no longer visible a few millimetres after the origin from the bladder neck. In the male, the preprostatic and the prostatic urethra are identifiable due to muscles that surround them. • Ischiatic tract: a perineal window is used (Fig. 16.1c). For the most proximal tract, the anal rosette can be used as an acoustic window (Fig. 16.1d). The ventral area of the rectum is where the urethra runs and is visible if dilated. • Penile tract (in males only): using a linear probe, the urethra can be followed from the perineal region to the penis tip. In all urethral tracts, transverse and longitudinal scans must be performed (Fig. 16.1e).

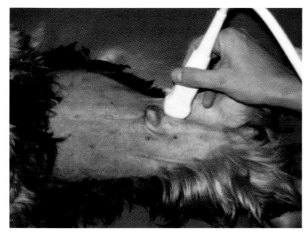

Figure 16.1a   Position 1, transverse scan of the bladder. In females, the midline just cranially to the pubis is taken as a reference point; in males, a parapreputial scan is used.

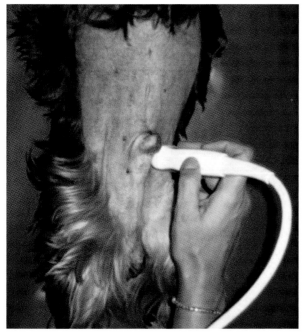

Figure 16.1b   Position 1: longitudinal scan of the bladder.

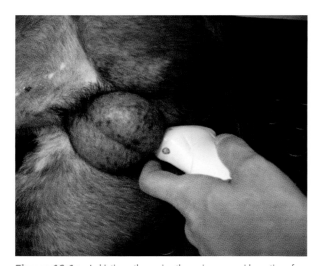

Figure 16.1c   Ischiatic urethra: using the perineum, a wide portion of the ischiatic urethra is identified.

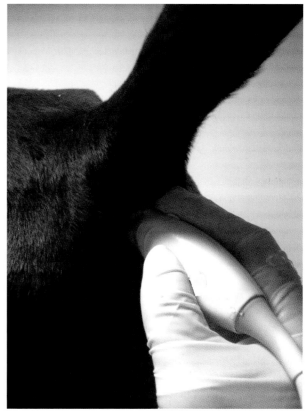

Figure 16.1d   Ischiatic urethra: it is identified using the anal rosette as acoustic window.

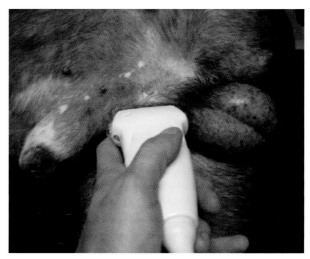

Figure 16.1e   Scan of the penile urethra.

ULTRASONOGRAPHIC ANATOMY – BLADDER (Fig. 16.2–5)

Location	• Middle-caudal abdomen.
Morphology and size	• Elongated and pear-shaped, variable according to the repletion degree.
Relationships with adjacent organs evaluable on ultrasonography	• Cranially: intestinal bundle. • Caudally: urethra. • Dorsally and laterally: uterus and descending colon. • Ventrally: mesenteric tissue, abdominal wall.

Wall	• Very variable parietal thickness depending on the repletion state (Fig. 16.2)
	  – Dog: from 1.4 (distended bladder) to 2.3 mm (not distended bladder)
	  – Cat: from 1.3 (distended bladder) to 1.7 mm (not distended bladder)
	     However, despite these values reported by literature, in large breed dogs the parietal thickness of an empty bladder can go up to 4 mm.
	• Ultrasonographic appearance of the wall: in most cases it is slightly hypoechoic compared to mesenteric tissue, and is uniform (Fig. 16.3). However, if distended, it can appear triple-layered (Fig. 16.4). Layers are very thin and are:
	  – Hyperechoic line: serous coat
	  – Hypoechoic layer: muscular coat
	  – Hyperechoic line: submucosa. The mucous coat is not distinguishable on ultrasonography.
	• Ureteral papillae: symmetrical parietal protrusions over the bladder trigone (Fig. 16.5).

Echostructure and echogenicity of the bladder content	• Homogeneous and anechoic content.
Tributary lymph nodes	• Iliac: lumbar and sacral.

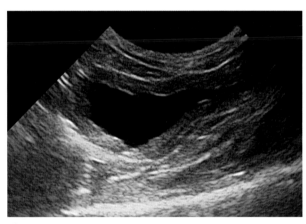

Figure 16.2 False parietal thickening in an empty bladder.

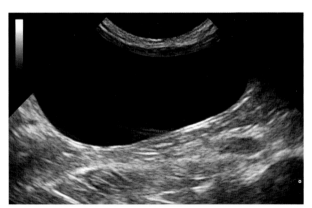

Figure 16.4 Distended bladder: the wall shows a fine stratigraphy (hyperechoic lumen-mucous coat interface, hypoechoic muscular coat, echoic serous coat).

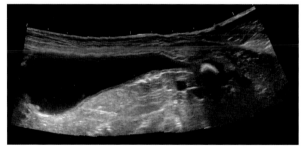

Figure 16.3 Longitudinal reconstruction of the normally repleted bladder of a bitch. Note the wall that is uniformly hypoechoic compared to surrounding tissues. Note the large stone (structure with hyperechoic interface associated with distal shadowing) in the urethra.

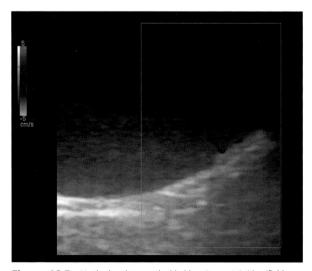

Figure 16.5 Urethral outlet over the bladder trigone. It is identifiable as a very small bulge in the trigone region. The Colour Doppler identifies the ureteral jet (urine flow from the ureter to the bladder).

ULTRASONOGRAPHIC ANATOMY – URETHRA (Fig. 16.6–8)

Location	• Caudal abdomen – perineal and penile region (male).
Morphology	• The urethra appears just a few millimetres caudally to the bladder neck as a linear structure with echoic regular wall. The lumen is visible only if dilated. The intrapelvic portion is not viewable due to overlapping pelvic bones (posterior shadowing artefact). The ischiatic urethra can be identified, especially in the male, and if dilated, through a perineal approach, using the anal rosette as an acoustic window (Fig. 16.6). In the male, the penile urethra runs inside a groove or cradle of the penile bone. In the cross section the cradle (Fig. 16.7) is identified and although differentiating the urethra as a structure is impossible, following its course is possible. In the longitudinal scan the penile bone surface, i.e. the urethra support, and the urethra if slightly distended are identified (Fig. 16.8).
Relationships with adjacent organs evaluable on ultrasonography	• Cranially: the bladder. • Dorsally, ventrally and laterally (male): the prostate (prostatic portion) and spongy bodies (penile portion). • Ventrally and laterally: penis bone and corpora cavernosa (penile portion).

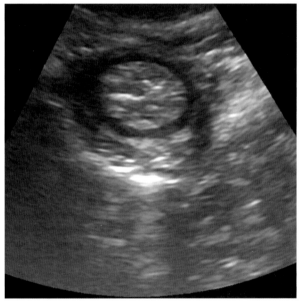

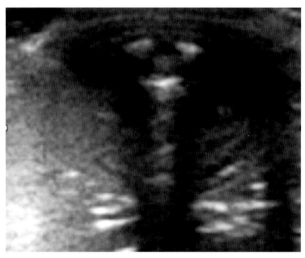

Figure 16.7 Transverse scan of the penile urethra: note the penile bone groove where the urethra runs.

Figure 16.6 Ischiatic urethra shown by a perineal window (anal rosette). Ventrally to the rectum the urethra is clearly visible in cross section, being slightly dilated in this patient.

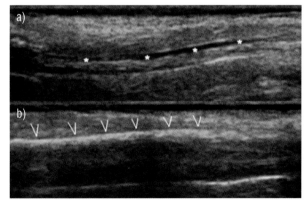

Figure 16.8 Longitudinal scan of the penile urethra. **a)** Image obtained dorsolaterally: the urethra without the penile bone is identified; asterisks indicate the hypoechoic lumen. **b)** Image obtained ventrally; the hyperechoic line made by the penile bone is identified (arrowheads).

ULTRASONOGRAPHIC CHANGES: BLADDER DISEASES

Bladder diseases can be classified into:

• Parietal abnormalities
• Bladder content abnormalities.

PARIETAL ABNORMALITIES

Bladder parietal diseases are essentially secondary to inflammatory (cystitis) or neoplastic infiltrates, or to traumatic events. To properly assess the wall, the bladder must be replete. A poorly distended bladder may mimic a false parietal thickening (Fig. 16.2).

CYSTITIS (Fig. 16.9)

Ultrasonographic findings:

- Thickened and irregular wall
- Location
  - Cranioventral: acute cystitis
  - Diffuse: chronic cystitis (Fig. 16.9)
- Gradual transition between diseased wall and 'normal' on ultrasonography wall
- Content: from normal (anechoic) to hyperechoic corpuscular; sometimes uroliths
- The parietal thickening does not cause occlusion of ureteral outlets.

In patients with chronic cystitis, aforementioned abnormalities tend to affect the whole wall. The gradual passage between diseased wall and normal on ultrasonography wall, associated to uroliths, is one key to differentiate on ultrasonography cystitis from bladder neoplasms (although in suspected cases, deeper investigations are needed).

POLYPOID CYSTITIS (FIG. 16.10)

It is a particular form of cystitis, with fleshy formations protruding into the bladder lumen. The differentiation with a neoplastic infiltrate is not always easy.

Ultrasonographic findings:

- Parietal thickening that features protruding polyps (narrow-base 'cauliflower-like' neoformations) in the bladder lumen (Fig. 16.10)
- Cranioventral or diffuse location
- The appearance can be consistent with neoplasms, but the final diagnosis is obtained by biopsy
- Often there are uroliths.

EMPHYSEMATOUS CYSTITIS (Fig. 16.11)

The emphysematous cystitis is a characteristic form of cystitis evaluable on ultrasonography by the intramural and, secondarily, even intraluminal gas. The gas is generated by bacteria (*E. coli, Proteus spp., Clostridium spp.*) more often found in animals with glycosuria.

Ultrasonographic findings:

- Cranioventral or diffuse parietal thickening
- Intramural and intraluminal gas (Fig. 16.11)
- Reverberation artefacts due to the pathological presence of bladder gas
- In cases with doubt, a subsidiary radiographic examination is useful.

NEOPLASM (Fig. 16.12)

The most common neoplasm is the transitional cell carcinoma followed by other epithelial or mesenchymal tumours (squamous cell carcinoma, lymphoma, fibrosarcoma, leiomyoma/sarcoma). Neoplastic bladder neoformations cause a pathological thickening of the wall, which usually shows a switchover (transition) clearly separated from the parietal portion normal 'on ultrasonography'.

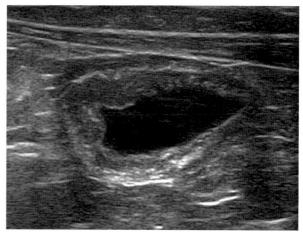

Figure 16.9 Chronic cystitis characterized by irregular and diffuse parietal thickening.

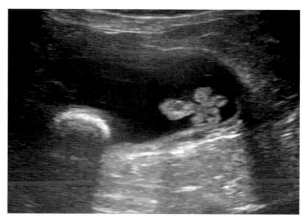

Figure 16.10 Bladder polyp in a dog with chronic cystitis. Note the urolith that probably caused the chronic cystitis (hyperechoic curved interface followed by posterior acoustic shadow).

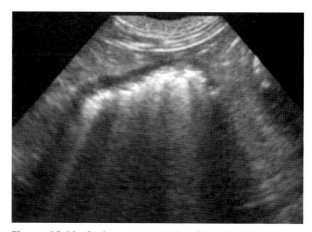

Figure 16.11 Emphysematous cystitis in a diabetic dog. The normal anechoic content of the bladder lumen is replaced by a hyperechoic interface that produces reverberation artefacts (gas). Some reverberations start from the bladder wall.

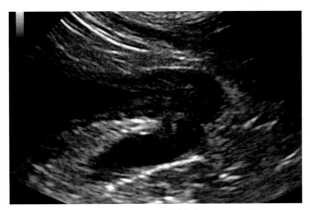

Figure 16.12 Parietal thickening in the bladder trigone region, associated with ureteral obstructive dilation: squamous cell carcinoma.

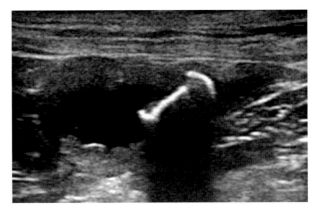

Figure 16.13 Bladder lithiasis associated with a picture of chronic cystitis in a nearly empty bladder.

ULTRASONOGRAPHIC FINDINGS:

- Large-base intramural neoformations
- Often protruding into the bladder lumen, sometimes eccentrically growing
- Location: usually, in the bladder neck or the bladder trigone
- Mixed echogenicity and echostructure; sometimes there are parenchymal mineralizations
- Possible ureteral or urethral obstruction, depending on the location of even very small masses (Fig. 16.12)
- Bladder neoplasms rarely diffusely invade the bladder wall.

Cytological examination through traumatic catheterization is preferable to transparietal cytology due to the risk of metastatic implant along the needle ride.

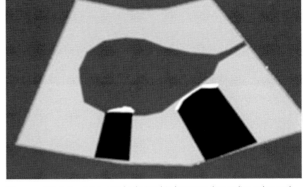

Figure 16.14 Anatomical relationship between descending colon and bladder: the closeness and similarity of artefacts could deceive a novice.

BLADDER CONTENTS ABNORMALITIES

Most common abnormalities of the bladder contents are stones, blood clots and urinary sediment.

CALCULOSIS (Fig. 16.13–14)

Ultrasonographic findings:

- Structures characterized by a hyperechoic interface, with well-defined edges, although often irregularly shaped (Fig. 16.13)
- Interfaces associated with clean posterior shadowing artefact
- Mobile elements, located in the bladder declivous portion
- Crystalluria: hyperechoic floating corpuscular content associated with absent or weak posterior shadowing.

The close anatomical relationship between descending colon and bladder and the reverberation artefact of the colic content can sometimes be misleading and mimic a bladder lithiasis (Fig. 16.14). In these situations, changing the probe orientation is appropriate using various scan angles or putting the patient in the quadrupedal posture. In case of lithiasis, the urolith will move by gravity into the ventral declivous portion of the bladder.

BLOOD CLOTS (Fig. 16.15)

They may be a result of traumas, cystitis, bladder haemorrhages and neoplasms.

Ultrasonographic findings:

- Generally echoic and mobile, floating in the bladder lumen (Fig. 16.15)
- Variable size and shape
- Lacking posterior shadowing.

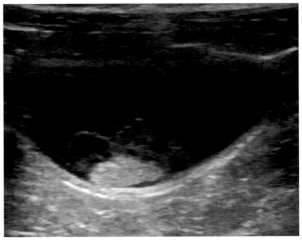

Figure 16.15 Typical appearance of a bladder clot.

SEDIMENT (Fig. 16.16)

With the patient in recumbency for some minutes at least, the sediment collects in the more declivous portion of the organ, forming a hyperechoic band that, depending on its composition, can produce a shadowing (Fig. 16.16a).

If the bladder is moved, the sediment is resuspended mixing with the anechoic urine. This is a way to differentiate a real sediment from a pseudo-sediment.

There are several types of bladder sediment with variable composition and echogenicity (Fig. 16.16).

TRAUMAS (Fig. 16.17)

Iatrogenic or traumatic events can cause bladder or urethral ruptures. In these situations, the ultrasonographic examination, often associated with a contrast radiographic examination, may provide important information on the bladder status and the trauma location and extension.

Ultrasonographic findings:

- Irregular wall; sometimes obvious parietal discontinuity areas (Fig. 16.17)
- Corpuscular and hyperechoic bladder content (haematuria)
- Bladder haematoma: floating endoluminal neoformation, irregular and predominantly hyperechoic
- Abdominal effusion (uroabdomen) and perivesical peritoneal reactivity.

The positive contrast radiology is the method of choice to diagnose a bladder rupture; nevertheless, injecting plenty of manually agitated saline through a catheter inserted in the bladder can be tried. Small air bubbles in the solution create some ultrasonographic contrast. The scan plane that is as aligned as possible with the utmost responsiveness of the perivesical mesentery is selected; then, it should be checked that the small hyperechoic bubbles do not pass in the peritoneum.

URETHRAL DISEASES

Typically, obstructive diseases require an ultrasonographic examination of the urethra. Most common causes include lithiasic, inflammatory or neoplastic processes.

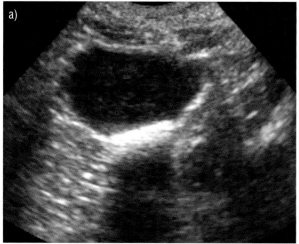

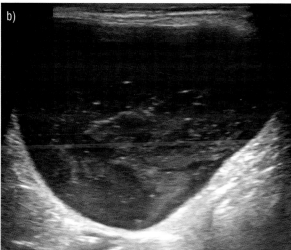

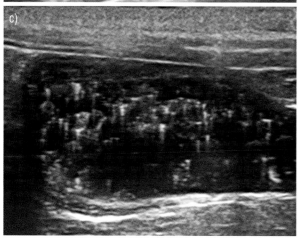

Figure 16.16 Different types of urinary sediment. **a)** Collected sediment forming a posterior acoustic shadow. This gives evidence that the sediment is mineralized. **b)** Suspended sediment. Particles are echoic, but in this case stating whether crystals are present is impossible. Once settled, the type of artefact can be evaluated. Echoic sediments without posterior shadowing are often associated with proteinic or cellular material. **c)** Suspended sediment generating reverberation artefacts that are air microbubbles. Some suspended lipid substances could mimic the same effect.

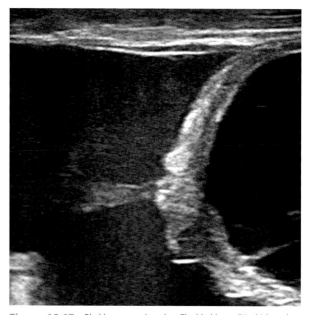

Figure 16.17 Bladder rupture in a dog. The bladder wall is thickened, there is an abdominal effusion and an echoic jet of material that flows out from the bladder lumen in the peritoneum.

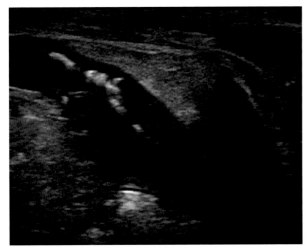

Figure 16.18 Parietal thickening of the bladder trigone region, associated with obstructive ureteral dilation: squamous cell carcinoma.

In cases of bladder overdistension, evaluating the explorable tract of the urethra (prepelvic, perineal and penile) is important; in cases with doubt, in suspected urethral ruptures, or if unable to evaluate the whole urethra, the ultrasonography must be associated to the contrast radiography.

NEOPLASM (Fig. 16.18)
The most common urethral neoplasm is the transitional cell carcinoma.

  Ultrasonographic findings:

- Irregular parietal thickening associated to injuries projecting in the urethral lumen (Fig. 16.18)
- Heterogeneous echostructure with predominantly hypoechoic appearance

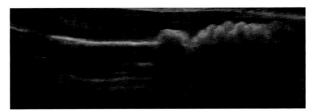

Figure 16.19 Penile urethra containing uroliths.

- Dystrophic mineralizations
- Possible extension and involvement of the bladder neck
- Tributary adenopathy.

LITHIASIS (Fig. 16.19)
- Hyperechoic structures with well-defined edges
- Associated with posterior shadowing artefact
- Urethral distension proximally to the obstruction.

RECOMMENDED READING

Petite A, Busoni V, Heinen MP, Billen F, Snaps F: Radiographic and ultra-sonographic findings of emphysematous cystitis in four nondiabetic dogs. Vet Radiol Ultrasound. 2006, 47(1): 90–93.

Benigni L, Lamb CR, Corzo-Menendez N, Holloway A, Eastwood JM: Lymphoma affecting the urinary bladder in three dogs and a cat. Vet Radiol Ultrasound. 2006, 47(5): 592–596.

Takiguchi M, Inaba M: Diagnostic ultrasound of polypoid cystitis in dogs. J Vet Med Sci. 2005, 67(1): 57–61.

Martinez I, Mattoon JS, Eaton KA, Chew DJ, DiBartola SP: Polypoid cystitis in 17 dogs (1978–2001). J Vet Intern Med. 2003, 17(4): 499–509.

Geisse AL, Lowry JE, Schaeffer DJ, Smith CW: Sonographic evaluation of urinary bladder wall thickness in normal dogs. Vet Radiol Ultrasound. 1997, 38(2): 132–137.

17 Adrenal glands

Gian Marco Gerboni

SCAN TECHNIQUE (Fig. 17.1)

Animal preparation	• 12 hours on an empty stomach, at least. • Wide hair-clipping, including last three intercostal spaces. • Dorsal recumbency, right lateral and left lateral.
Probes	• Microconvex, 7.5 MHz mean frequency for dogs <10 kg, 5 MHz mean frequency for large breed/obese dogs. • Linear, high frequency (7.5–10 MHz) for small breed animals and cats.
Scans and respective probe position 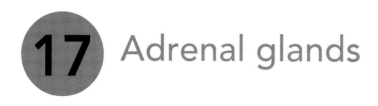	**LEFT ADRENAL GLAND** • Longitudinal scan (position 3, Fig. 17.1a): the probe is placed perpendicular to the skin surface, the ultrasound beam is aligned perpendicularly to the aorta, which is followed caudocranially up to the renal artery emersion (recognizable by the characteristic hook shape). The adrenal gland is located in the adipose tissue between the renal artery (caudally), and cranial mesenteric and celiac arteries (cranially), which form a pair of vessels always well recognizable. To visualize it in its longitudinal axis, slightly rotating the probe clockwise is often necessary, since it is not perfectly parallel to the aorta. In the long axis, the left adrenal gland appears with an '8' (or peanut) shape. Best images are obtained when the kidney is not included in the scan plane and the gland is as superficial as possible on the scan plane. • Transverse scan (position 3): the probe is perpendicular to the skin surface, the beam is transversely oriented by 90° to the long axis; the adrenal gland appears with an oval or triangular shape. • Intercostal scans (position 4): occasionally used to search for the adrenal gland over the 12th intercostal space. **RIGHT ADRENAL GLAND** • Longitudinal scan (position 10, Fig. 17.1b): the probe is placed perpendicularly to the skin surface, the ultrasound beam is aligned parallel to the caudal vena cava, cranially to the hilum of the right kidney. After the caudal vena cava is localized, the probe is slightly moved laterally (towards the kidney), maintaining the parallelism with the vena cava. In the long axis, the adrenal gland appears with an arrow or comma shape, with a thinner caudal pole and a more expanded cranial pole. Note that using a right side scan is almost always possible to identify both the right adrenal gland and the left adrenal gland. To avoid any mistakes, the renal artery and cranial mesenteric/celiac arteries can be used as landmarks. Following the aorta and proceeding in the caudocranial direction, the renal artery, the left adrenal gland, and the origin of cranial mesenteric artery and celiac arteries (approximately at the cranial pole of the right kidney) are identified. Then, the probe is tilted ventrally towards the vena cava and the right adrenal gland is identified. In any case, the right adrenal gland is always cranial to the origin of cranial mesenteric and celiac arteries. Best images are obtained when the kidney is not in the scan field (see also Fig. 6.5, Chapter 6). • Transverse scan (position 10): the probe is perpendicular to the skin surface, the beam is transversely oriented by 90° to the long axis; the adrenal gland appears with an oval or triangular shape. • Intercostal scans (position 9): occasionally used to search for the adrenal gland over the 12th intercostal space. This scan is very helpful, especially in middle/large-size breed dogs when applying enough pressure from the retrocostal position is impossible.

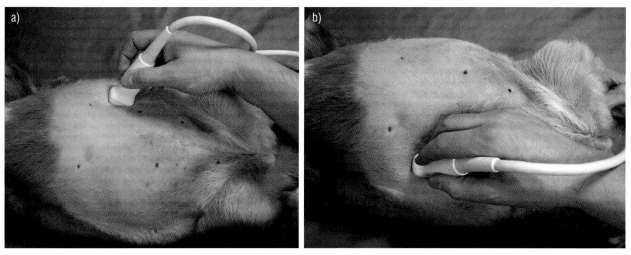

Figure 17.1 Probe positions to scan the adrenal glands. **a)** Positions 3–4. Longitudinal scan of the left adrenal gland. Microconvex probe. **b)** Position 10. Longitudinal scan of the right adrenal gland. Microconvex probe.

ULTRASONOGRAPHIC ANATOMY (Fig. 17.2–7)

Location	• Left and right cranial abdomen.
Morphology	**LEFT ADRENAL GLAND** • Dog: bilobate and elongated shape, with symmetrical cranial and caudal pole, and a thinner central isthmus, giving a '8' or peanut shape. • Cat: oval-shaped. **RIGHT ADRENAL GLAND** • Dog: triangular or arrow shape; the cranial pole is shorter and wider compared to the caudal pole. • Cat: oval-shaped.
Relationships with adjacent organs evaluable on ultrasonography	**LEFT ADRENAL GLAND** • Cranially: mesenteric artery and celiac artery. • Laterally: cranial pole of the left kidney. • Medially: descending aorta. • Caudally: left renal artery. **RIGHT ADRENAL GLAND** • Cranially: caudate lobe of the liver. • Laterally: right kidney. • Medially: caudal vena cava. • Caudally: emersion of celiac and caudal mesenteric arteries.
Size	There are various ways to assess the adrenal gland's size; the most useful is possibly to measure the caudal pole of the gland (Barthez et al. 1998), which is reported in the following normal ranges: • Dog: normal diameter between 3.5 and 7.4 mm • Cat: normal diameter between 2.8 and 4.3 mm The most recent literature (Hoerauf et al., 1999; Choi et al. 2011) provides other ranges in dogs: • <3 mm: hypoplasia • 3–6.5 mm: Normal • 6.6 to 7.4 mm: simple hyperplasia (stress and non-endocrine diseases) • >7.5 mm: hyperplasia due to suspected hyperadrenocorticism **NOTE:** • The literature reports higher variability ranges, and a number of concomitant diseases can affect the adrenal glands' sizes. • A percentage of patients with hyperadrenocorticism may have normal-sized adrenal glands. • The adrenal glands ultrasonographic evaluation must always be combined with the clinical and laboratory picture, and never taken as the only discriminatory factor.
Edges	• Thin, smooth and rounded.

(Continued →)

ULTRASONOGRAPHIC ANATOMY (continued)

Echogenicity	• Thin echoic capsule (visible only if the ultrasound beam is exactly perpendicular). • Hypoechoic outer cortex. • Hyperechoic inner medullary. • The differentiation between the cortex and the medullary echogenicity is not always obvious. • Overall, they are isoechoic compared to the renal cortex. • Hypoechoic compared to the retroperitoneal adipose tissue. • The differentiation between the cortex and the medullary is sometimes visible in dogs, and requires a high-frequency probe. The cortico-medullary differentiation is rarely observed in cats; on the contrary, especially in elderly animals, finding mineralization foci is common, which must be considered incidental findings with no clinical significance if not combined with other gland changes (Fig. 17.6 and 17.7).
Echostructure	• Mean. • Homogeneous, both for the cortex and the medullary.
Vessels	Phrenicoabdominal vein • It runs ventrally to the gland in the central portion. Phrenicoabdominal artery • It runs dorsally to the gland in the central portion (only visible if the Colour Doppler method is used).
Tributary lymph nodes	Lumboaortic (identifiable only if pathological).

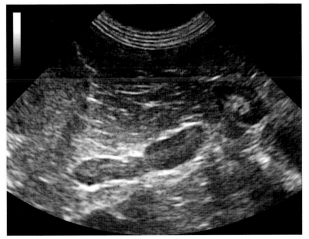

Figure 17.2 Longitudinal scan of the normal left adrenal gland. The image shows the characteristic '8' or 'peanut' shape.

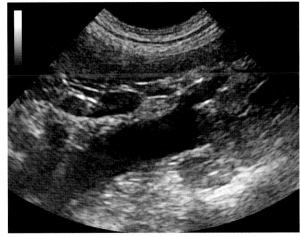

Figure 17.4 Longitudinal scan of the left adrenal gland. Vascular landmarks of the left adrenal gland region are identified: cranially to the cranial pole, mesenteric and celiac arteries; dorsally, the aorta artery; caudally to the gland, the renal artery.

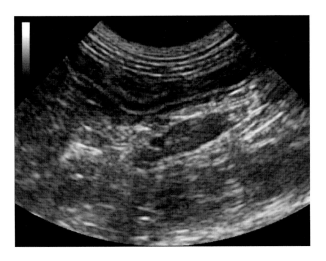

◀ **Figure 17.3** Longitudinal scan of the normal right adrenal gland. The image shows the shortest size of the cranial pole and, ventrally to the gland, the phrenicoabdominal vein in cross section.

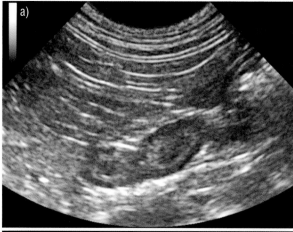

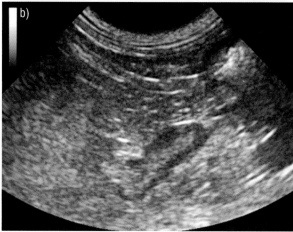

Figure 17.5   Normal ultrasonographic appearance of left **(a)** and right **(b)** adrenal glands in the longitudinal scan. The gland features the thin hyperechoic capsule, the hypoechoic cortex and the hyperechoic medullary compared to the cortex.

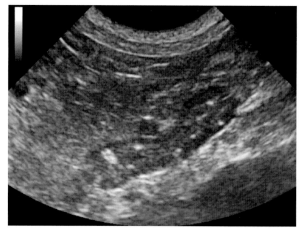

Figure 17.6   Left adrenal gland. Disseminated mineralizations of the gland parenchyma not associated with adrenomegaly.

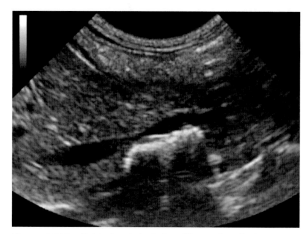

Figure 17.7   Right adrenal gland of an older cat; the reflective acoustic interface and the posterior acoustic shadowing indicate the gland's complete mineralization.

ULTRASONOGRAPHIC CHANGES

Main ultrasonographic changes of adrenal glands		
	Bilateral and uniform symmetrical changes	**Unilateral or bilateral asymmetrical changes**
Increased volume	Simple hyperplasia Nodular hyperplasia Pituitary hyperadrenocorticism (pituitary Cushing) Pituitary hyperadrenocorticism under treatment with trilostane	Non-secreting neoplasms, Secreting neoplasms (e.g. adrenal Cushing) Rarely, haematomas Abscesses Cysts Granulomas
Volume reduction	Hypoplasia secondary to corticosteroids (iatrogenic Cushing) Addison's disease hypoplasia	Hypoplasia secondary to a secreting-corticosteroids contralateral neoplasm (adrenal Cushing)

BILATERAL AND UNIFORM SYMMETRIC CHANGES (Fig. 17.8–12)

SIMPLE HYPERPLASIA

Adrenal glands increase in volume as a result of 'stress' factors or in non-endocrine diseases.

Hyperplastic glands are characterized by:

- Preserved shape
- Increased sizes (caudal pole diameter >6.5 mm)
- Normal to reduced echogenicity
- Normal echostructure.

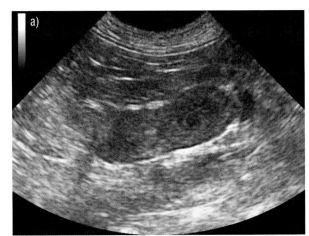
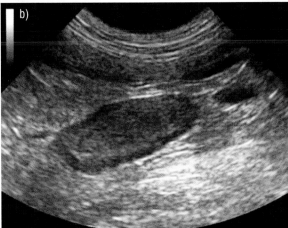
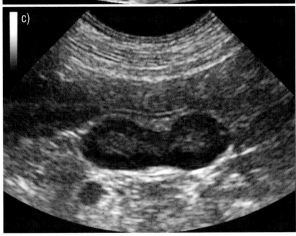

Figure 17.8 a, b, c In hyperplastic adrenal glands the shape is preserved but the gland appears more rounded and hypoechoic, and the cortex thickness can vary considerably.

PITUITARY HYPERPLASIA AND HYPERADRENOCORTICISM

The pituitary hyperadrenocorticism is the most common cause of Cushing's syndrome in dogs and cats (approximately 80–85 per cent of cases). Adrenal glands undergo a symmetrical and bilateral change in shape and increase in size.

In 95 per cent of cases it is a simple cortex hyperplasia, characterized by:

- Preserved shape with more rounded edges
- Increased sizes (caudal pole diameter >7.4 mm)
- Reduced echogenicity
- Echostructure within normal limits, thickened cortex easily distinguishable from the medullary
- Associated injuries (changes secondary to hyperadrenocorticism, infiltrative liver disease, diffuse mineralizations)

In a certain percentage of patients with hyperadrenocorticism, adrenal glands may be normal; so this diagnosis should not

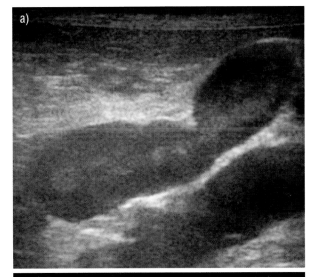
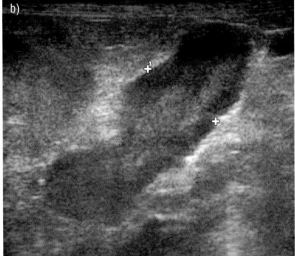

Figure 17.9 Left adrenal gland **(a)** and right adrenal gland **(b)** of a dog. Bilateral adrenal hyperplasia secondary to pituitary hyperadrenocorticism. The shape of the left and right glands is normal, poles appear rounded, and the diameter measured at the caudal pole is greater than 7.5 mm.

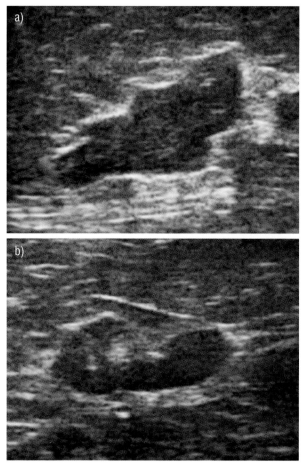

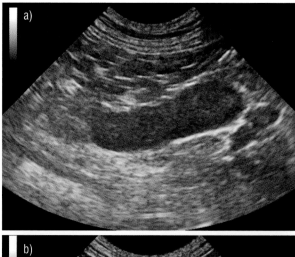

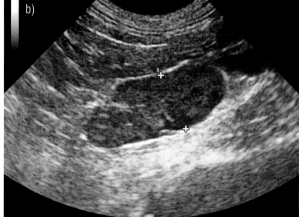

Figure 17.10 Right adrenal gland **(a)** and left adrenal gland **(b)** of a dog. Nodular adrenal hyperplasia secondary to pituitary hyperadrenocorticism. The shape and profile of the right adrenal gland are changed by small nodular structures that increase its volume; even the left gland is increased in size.

Figure 17.11 Left adrenal gland **(a)** and right adrenal gland **(b)**. Bilateral adrenal hyperplasia in a dog with pituitary hyperadrenocorticism and treated with trilostane. The gland's size continues to increase during the therapy; note that the right gland measured at the caudal pole is 13.1 mm in diameter.

be excluded if clinical and laboratory findings are indicative of Cushing's. In these cases, performing serial ultrasonographic check-ups is useful.

NODULAR HYPERPLASIA

In 5 per cent of cases, the bilateral cortex hyperplasia may be nodular; nevertheless, it is a less common variation of the pituitary hyperadrenocorticism. In these cases, ultrasonographic findings are similar to an early-stage neoplasm:

- Preserved shape with more rounded and irregular edges
- Increased sizes (caudal pole diameter >7.4 mm)
- Reduced echogenicity
- Heterogeneous cortex echostructure due to small nodular structures.

PITUITARY HYPERADRENOCORTICISM IN TRILOSTANE TREATED ANIMALS (MANTIS 2003)

- In serial checkups, adrenal glands increase in size
- The cortex becomes more hypoechoic

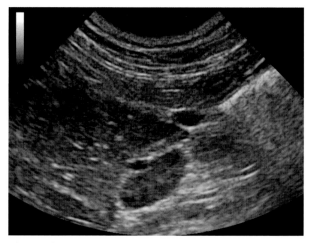

Figure 17.12 Longitudinal scan of the right adrenal gland in a cat; the gland is hyperplastic with a rounded shape; ventrally, the phrenicoabdominal vein is highlighted.

- The medullary becomes more hyperechoic
- Increased corticomedullary contrast
- In the aforementioned study, three of 19 patients showed a distortion of the glandular echostructure.

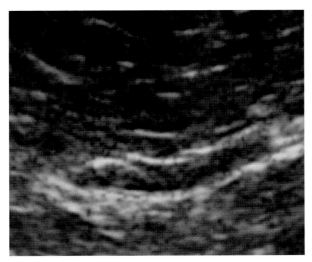

Figure 17.13 Longitudinal scan of the hypoplastic left adrenal gland in a dog with Addison's disease. The gland retains the typical shape, the phrenicoabdominal vein that runs ventrally is well clear, but thickness and diameter of poles is significantly reduced.

HYPOPLASIA AND HYPOADRENOCORTICISM (Fig. 17.13)

The adrenal gland's volume decreases during treatments with corticosteroids, because they inhibit the hypothalamus–pituitary–adrenal axis, or in cases of hypoadrenocorticism.

The gland atrophy observed in patients with Addison's disease is highlighted by:

- Preserved shape with more sharp edges
- Reduced size, length and thickness (caudal pole diameter <3 mm)
- Echogenicity within normal limits
- Echostructure within normal limits; the corticomedullary distinction is more difficult to identify.

UNILATERAL OR BILATERAL ASYMMETRICAL CHANGES (Fig. 17.14–18)

Haematomas, abscesses, cysts and granulomas are rare but possible changes of one or both glands. The non-neoplastic

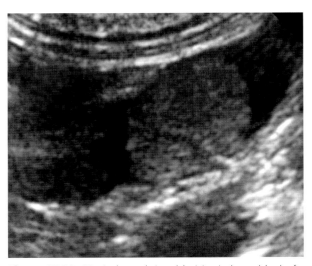

Figure 17.14 Massive hyperechoic nodular injury in the caudal pole of the left adrenal gland.

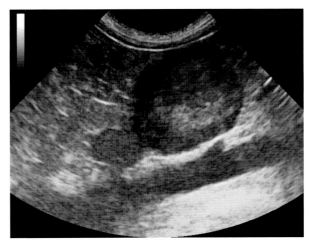

Figure 17.15 A massive nodule with non-uniform echostructure deforming the caudal pole of the left adrenal gland. The distal field shows the longitudinal course of the aorta.

adrenal masses determine changes in shape, size and echostructure, of all or a part of the gland.

By an ultrasonographic point of view, a non-neoplastic solid neoformation is not distinguishable from a neoplasm, although the second option is statistically much more likely.

NEOPLASMS

The most represented adrenal neoplasms in small animals are cortical adenoma, cortical carcinoma, medullary pheochromocytoma and, more rarely, metastasis of other neoplasms. Adrenal neoplasms can be secreting or non-secreting. About 20 per cent of Cushing's syndrome cases are caused by an adrenal neoplasm (adenoma or carcinoma). Pheochromocytomas can produce catecholamines.

Consistent clinical and/or laboratory findings gear towards a specific condition. However, the diagnosis of adrenal injury (nodule or mass) can be incidental, not associated with clinical or lab tests changes. In these cases, possible causes include a non-secreting neoplasm or a non-neoplastic injury. Especially if the injury is small, the definitive diagnosis is impossible with ultrasonography alone. In these cases, ultrasonographic check-ups (every some week) may be useful to assess the evolution. Ultrasonographic features that point to a diagnosis of malignant adrenal neoplasm are:

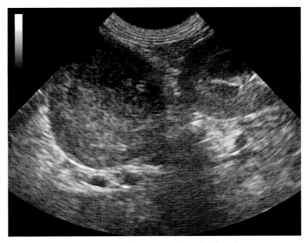

Figure 17.16 Right adrenal mass in a dog with adrenal hyperadrenocorticism. Dorsally to the mass, mesenteric and celiac arteries are visualized; caudally, the cranial pole of the left kidney is shown.

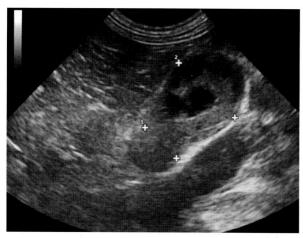

Figure 17.17 Adrenomegaly of the left adrenal gland with non-uniform and microcystic echostructure of the caudal pole.

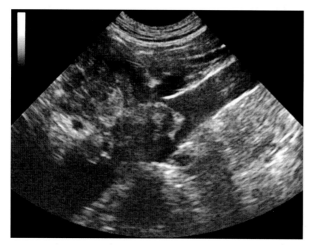

Figure 17.18 Right adrenal mass characterized by non-uniform echostructure and metastatic invasion of the caudal vena cava lumen; the image shows the partial occlusion created by the echoic and projecting structure.

- Localized or generalized loss of the normal shape
- Increased size (diameter >40 mm is considered a malignancy character)
- Isoechoic-hypoechoic or hyperechoic heterogeneous echostructure with hyperechoic foci and posterior acoustic shadowing
- Irregular capsule and edges

- Invasion of surrounding structures, in particular vessels, kidneys and liver. The vascular invasion usually involves the phrenicoabdominal vein and, through this one, the caudal vena cava. More rarely, renal vessels are involved (vein and artery) or the aorta
- The pheochromocytoma is reported to be more often homogeneous and hypoechoic, and rarely mineralized (about 10 per cent of cases)
- In epithelial neoplasms, calcifications can be found in 30–50 per cent of cases.

If the adrenal neoplasm secretes corticosteroids (adrenal hyperadrenocorticism), the following ultrasonographic findings can be observed:

- Hypoplasia of the contralateral adrenal gland secondary to suppression of the hypothalamus–pituitary–adrenal axis
- Steroid liver disease characterized by hepatomegaly with increased parenchymal echogenicity and homogeneous echostructure. These features are associated with a glycogen liver accumulation
- Sediment in the biliary tract; sometimes intrahepatic cholestasis
- Diffuse mineralizations (kidney, spleen)
- Bladder distension; the bladder becomes piriform (typical of PU/PD patients)
- Venous or arterial thrombosis secondary to hypercoagulability.

RECOMMENDED READING

Combes A, Vandermeulen E, Duchateau L, Peremans K, Daminet S, Saunders JH. Ultrasonographic measurements of adrenal glands in cats with hyperthyroidism. Vet Radiol Ultrasound. 2012; 53(2): 210–216.

Pey P, Daminet S, Smets PMY, Duchateau L, Travetti O, Saunders JH. Effect of glucocorticoid administration on adrenal gland size and sonographic appearance in beagle dogs. Vet Radiol Ultrasound. 2012; 53(2): 204–209.

Choi J, Kim H, Yoon J: Ultrasonographic adrenal gland measurements in clinically normal small breed dogs and comparison with pituitary-dependent hyperadrenocorticism. J Vet Med Sci, 2011; 73(8): 985–989.

Mantis P, Lamb CR, Witt AL, Neiger R: Changes in ultrasonographic appearance of adrenal glands in dogs with pituitary-dependent hyperadrenocorticism treated with trilostane. Veterinary Radiology & Ultrasound 2003; 44(6): 682–685.

Moore LE, Biller DS, Smith TA. Use of abdominal Ultrasonography in the diagnosis of primary hyperaldosteronism in a cat. J Am Vet Med Assoc. 2000; 217: 213–215.

Barthez PY, Nyland TG, Feldman EC. Ultrasonographic evaluation of adrenal glands in dogs. J Am Vet Med Assoc 1998; 207: 1180–1183.

18 Neck region ultrasonography

Gian Marco Gerboni

SCAN TECHNIQUE (Fig. 18.1–3)

Animal preparation	• Wide hair-clipping of the neck, from the angle of the mandible to the chest entrance. • Dorsal recumbency, right and left lateral recumbency, sternal position.
Probes	• Linear, high frequency (7.5–15 MHz)
Scans and respective probe position	• Dorsal scan: the probe is positioned laterally to the neck, in the most cranial portion, to examine salivary glands, the parotid gland and retromandibular lymph nodes (Fig. 18.1a). • Transverse scan: the probe is positioned in a transverse plane to the centre of the neck, in contact with the base of the tongue and larynx, to examine lymph nodes, the larynx, the trachea, the esophagus, the thyroid, parathyroid glands and vessels (Fig. 18.1b). • Longitudinal scan: the probe is positioned along the longitudinal axis of the neck, to examine the trachea, the esophagus, the thyroid and parathyroid glands, vascular structures and lymph nodes (Fig. 18.1c).

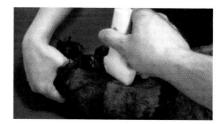

Figure 18.1a Dorsal recumbency and dorsal scan of the neck region. With the probe positioned laterally to the neck, in the most cranial portion salivary glands, the parotid gland and retromandibular lymph nodes are examined.

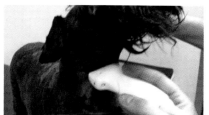

Figure 18.1b A patient in sternal position or quadrupedal posture. Transverse scan with the probe positioned at the centre of the neck, in contact with the base of the tongue, then the larynx and finally the trachea. Vascular structures, lymph nodes, the larynx, the trachea, thyroid glands and parathyroid glands are examined.

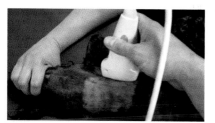

Figure 18.1c The dorsal recumbency allows for a more comfortable position for the operator, but is not always tolerated by the patient. The probe leans on the jugular furrow for a longitudinal scan of the thyroid gland, vascular structures and ipsilateral parathyroid glands. Using high-frequency linear probes is recommended.

ULTRASONOGRAPHIC ANATOMY - SALIVARY GLANDS (Fig. 18.2–3)

Location	• Cervical region in the more cranial portion, caudally to the angle of the mandible for the mandibular gland. • Rostral to the ear canal for the parotid gland.
Organs evaluable on ultrasonography	• The mandibular salivary gland appears superficially and rostrally to the convergence between the linguofacial and the maxillary veins. • The parotid salivary gland is oriented vertically and rostrally to the ear canal.
Morphology	• The mandibular salivary gland is oval, rounded or triangular in shape, surrounded by a thin hyperechoic capsule (Fig. 18.2). • The parotid salivary gland is thin and less defined, more irregular and hypoechoic compared to the mandibular salivary gland, mainly due to the limited thickness and more pronounced lobulation (Fig. 18.3).
Size	• Subjective evaluation.
Edges	• Thin, smooth and regular.
Echogenicity	• Mandibular: hyperechoic compared to the digastric muscle; the centre shows fine echoic striae that define the gland hilum. • Parotid gland: isoechoic compared to surrounding muscles.
Echostructure	• Mandibular gland: fine and homogeneous; typical echostructure of the glandular tissue. • Parotid gland: more heterogeneous; much like the muscle tissue that surrounds it.

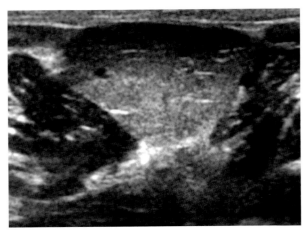

Figure 18.2 Typical appearance of the salivary gland: well-defined, fine and hyperechoic compared to surrounding muscle structures.

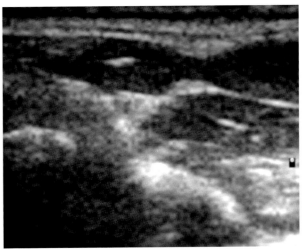

Figure 18.3 Parotid: ill-defined, isoechoic compared to the surrounding muscle tissue; it differs due to the different echostructure (the parotid gland lacks the classic muscle striae).

LYMPH NODES

Location	• Cranial cervical region in the more cranial portion, caudally to the angle of the mandible.
Organs evaluable on ultrasonography	• Mandibular lymph nodes, two–three per side, are located medially and caudally to mandibular salivary glands. • Retropharyngeal lymph nodes, dorsal to the pharynx and medial to mandibular salivary glands. • Superficial cervical lymph nodes located in the neck muscles fascia, and deep cervical lymph nodes located laterally and ventrally to the trachea.
Morphology	• Oval or ellipsoidal in shape.
Size	• 5–10 mm in length for mandibular lymph nodes. • 20–40 mm in length for retropharyngeal lymph nodes.
Echogenicity	• Hypoechoic compared to the surrounding adipose tissue. • Isoechoic compared to salivary glands.
Echostructure	• Homogeneous, fine.

LARYNX (Fig. 18.4–5)

Location	• Cranial cervical region, in the ventral portion of the neck on the median plane.
Organs evaluable on ultrasonography	• It is located caudally to the tongue and connects the lower portion of the pharynx to the trachea.
Morphology and echostructure	• In the cross section it is triangular, because its most cranial portion is bounded by thyroid cartilages, while the most caudal portion is bounded by cricoid cartilages. In dogs and cats, vocal processes of arytenoid cartilages are identifiable as two dorsal echoic lines, parallel to the probe (Fig. 18.4). • In the longitudinal section, the epiglottis is identifiable as a short echoic line parallel to the probe and dorsal to the cranial portion of the thyroid cartilage.
Normal motion	• Lateral abduction of vocal processes during the inspiration and return to the starting position during expiration (Fig. 18.5).

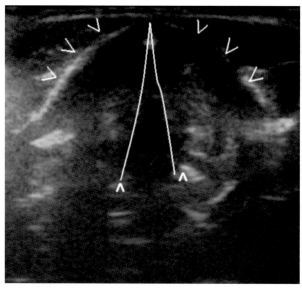

Figure 18.4 Transverse scan of the larynx of a dog over vocal ligaments (white lines) that join vocal processes (∧∧). Thyroid cartilages (∨∨) delimit it, giving the larynx the classic triangular shape.

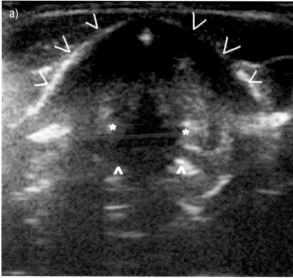

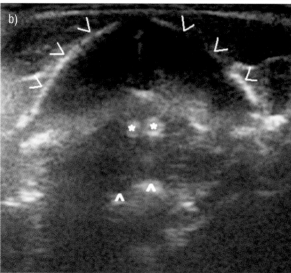

Figure 18.5 **a)** Inspiration: vocal processes (∧∧) are abducted laterally. **b)** Expiration: vocal processes (∨∨) return to their original position.

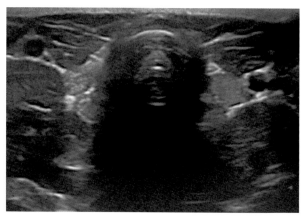

Figure 18.6a Transverse scan of the ventral cervical region of a dog. Just caudally to the larynx, the trachea is recognizable by its shape and reverberation artefacts. Laterally, both on the right and left, carotid arteries are recognizable (spherical anechoic structures). Between the trachea and the carotid artery, thyroid lobes are visible in the transverse scan.

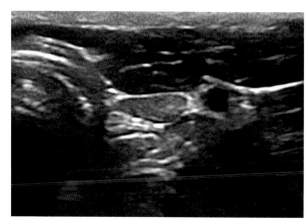

Figure 18.6b Transverse scan of the left thyroid lobe. Starting from **Figure 18.6a**, as soon as the thyroid lobe is identified, ultrasonographic device parameters (zoom, contrast, depth) are adjusted to enhance the image. The left thyroid lobe has a triangular shape, is a fine echostructure, is hyperechoic compared to surrounding muscle tissues and is limited by a thin hyperechoic capsule.

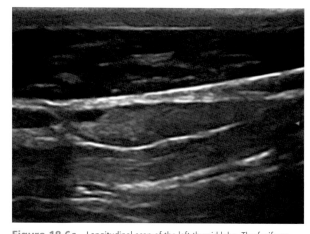

Figure 18.6c Longitudinal scan of the left thyroid lobe. The fusiform gland is characterized by a fine echostructure, and a hyperechoic parenchyma compared to surrounding muscle structures. It is delimited by a thin hyperechoic capsule. Note the cranial or external parathyroid gland, rounded and hypoechoic. In most superficial planes, sternocephalic and sternothyroid muscles can be identified, while in distal and deeper fields the longus capitis and the longus colli muscles are visualized.

THYROID (Fig. 18.6)

Location	• Cranial cervical region, in the ventral portion of the neck, at the second tracheal ring, just caudally to the larynx.
Organs evaluable on ultrasonography	• Right and left thyroid lobes: starting from a transverse scan, the larynx is identified (on palpation it is recognized by the triangular shape); then, slightly caudally, the trachea is identified as a circular structure containing air and located on the median plane. • Over first tracheal rings, carotid arteries located laterally to the trachea are searched for (Fig. 18.6a). • Thyroid lobes are delimited by the trachea medially, and carotid arteries laterally (Fig. 18.6b). • After their identification on the transverse plane, the probe is rotated by 90 degrees to obtain the longitudinal scan (Fig. 18.6c).
Morphology	• In the longitudinal section, lobes are fusiform or ellipsoidal, surrounded by a thin capsule. • In the cross-section, they appear round or triangular.
Size	Dog, normal size: • 25–30 mm in length. • 4–6 mm in diameter. Cat, normal size: • 18–22 mm in length. • 2.5–4 mm in diameter. Volume: it can be calculated using the formula $V = pi/6 \times (L \times T \times H)$. (V: volume in mm^3; pi/6 = 3.14/6 = 0.52; L = length in mm; T = thickness in mm; H = height in mm). The normal volume is related to the weight and the body surface area. Obviously, the measurement of these values is affected by a variability linked to the observer. • Most notably the length measurement can compromise the reproducibility.
Edges	• Thin and regular.
Echogenicity	• Isoechoic compared to the surrounding tissue and slightly hyperechoic compared to cervical muscles.
Echostructure	• Homogeneous. • Occasionally non-uniform with hypoechoic-hyperechoic foci.
Vessels	• The cranial and caudal thyroid artery and vein are only distinguishable using the Doppler.

PARATHYROID GLANDS (Fig. 18.7)

Location	• Cranial cervical region, in the ventral portion of the neck.
Organs evaluable on ultrasonography	• Cranial and caudal parathyroid glands (left and right) (Fig. 18.7). • The two cranial glands are located in the extrathyroidal fascia at the cranial pole of thyroid glands. • The two caudal glands are located within the parenchyma of the caudal pole of thyroid glands. • Additional and/or ectopic parathyroid glands are a possible finding.
Morphology	• Ellipsoidal in shape.
Size	Dog, normal size: • 3.3 mm in length. • 2 mm in diameter. • However, they are highly variable and often not visible in a large breed dog (healthy), while they are visible in a small breed dog.
Edges	• Thin and regular.
Echogenicity	• Hypoechoic or anechoic.
Echostructure	• Homogeneous, delimited by a thin invisible capsule

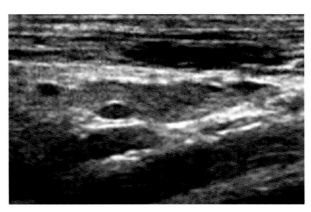

Figure 18.7 Longitudinal scan of a thyroid lobe in a normal dog. Within the thyroid lobe structure, parathyroid glands are visible and identifiable as two anechoic, oval, well-defined structures, one adjacent to the cranial pole and the other located within the body.

MOST COMMON SALIVARY GLANDS DISEASES OF ULTRASONOGRAPHIC INTEREST

SIALOCELE (Fig. 18.8)
- Often secondary to previous inflammations or traumas, to sialoliths or a neoplasm affecting the salivary duct opening
- They are identified as wide collections of fluid material rich in hyperechoic foci which extend ventrally, but have one side of contact at least with the salivary gland (Fig. 18.8)
- Often, the capsule is not visible in zones of contact
- Sometimes a dilated and injured duct is identifiable.

SIALOLITHS
- They are mineral collections occluding the salivary gland duct
- A sialocele is identified
- The sialolith can be identified but the radiology is more sensitive and specific, especially using a contrast agent.

For changes of regional lymph nodes, see Chapter 10.

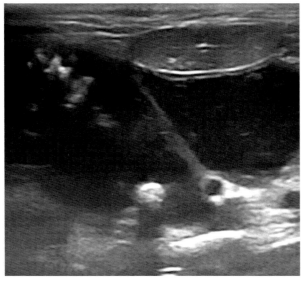

Figure 18.8 Sialocele of the mandibular gland. Superficially, the mandibular gland protrudes on a collection that is fluid but rich of echoic material.

LARYNX ULTRASONOGRAPHIC CHANGES

Most common laryngeal diseases of ultrasonographic interest can be classified as:

- Inflammatory
- Functional
- Neoplastic.

Sometimes, functional changes may be due to a chronic inflammatory process.

LARYNGITIS
- Ultrasonographic findings are often non-specific and must be correlated to the clinical symptomatology
- Thickening and hyperechogenicity of vocal ligaments
- Thickening of laryngeal and tracheal walls.

LARYNGEAL PARALYSIS (Fig. 18.9)
- The laryngeal paralysis can be unilateral or bilateral; the ultrasonography enables one to visualize cuneiform processes and vocal cords, to evaluate the motion periodicity and symmetry
- The diagnostic criteria of the laryngeal paralysis are reduction and asymmetry of the vocal cords motion
- In the laryngeal paralysis, the motion of arytenoid cartilages is no longer an abduction, but becomes dorsoventral due to contraction of cricothyroid muscles (up and down) (Fig. 18.9).

LARYNGEAL MASSES (Fig. 18.10)
In the literature, the lymphoma, the squamous cell carcinoma and the adenocarcinoma are most common laryngeal neoplasms in cats, while the carcinoma and the adenocarcinoma are most common laryngeal neoplasms in dogs. Primarily in cats, benign neoformations are also reported; they are often echoic and related to hyperplasias and metaplasias secondary to chronic inflammations.

Laryngeal masses tend to be hypoechoic, therefore not easily identifiable, especially in cats that have a fully anechoic larynx except for vocal processes.

- The delimiting surrounding gas helps to identify them (Fig. 18.10)
- The changed laryngeal symmetry, the anatomical variation or the dislocation of the central air column allow one to identify the mass effect associated.

THYROID GLAND ULTRASONOGRAPHIC CHANGES

CANINE HYPOTHYROIDISM (Fig. 18.11)
The ultrasonography of thyroid glands can be used to diagnose a primary hypothyroidism and/or differentiate it from the 'euthyroid sick syndrome'. Ultrasonographic features detectable in hypothyroidism are:

- Rounded edges in the transverse scan, with loss of the triangular shape (Fig. 18.11a)
- Reduced volume (Fig. 18.11b)
- Decreased echogenicity compared to the sternothyroid muscle

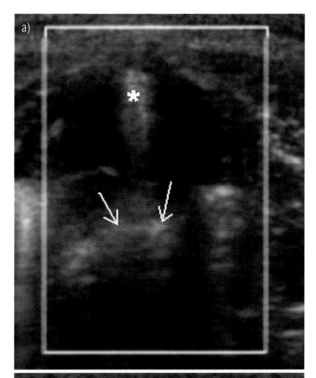

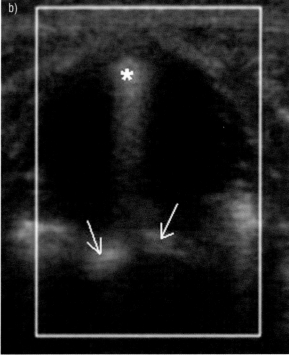

Figure 18.9 A patient with laryngeal paralysis; transverse scans of the larynx over vocal cords and vocal processes obtained during respiration. Vocal processes (indicated by arrows) undergo dorsal (up, Fig. 18.9a) and ventral (down, Fig. 18.9b) movements, but no lateral movements (as it should normally be). The air column (*) is reduced in size, both during inspiration and expiration.

- Non-uniform echostructure with diffuse small nodular injuries
- Irregular capsule
- Changes visualized in two lobes may be different
- The dog with 'euthyroid sick syndrome' has thyroid lobes with normal ultrasonographic features.

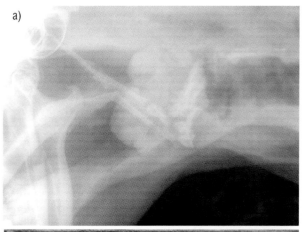

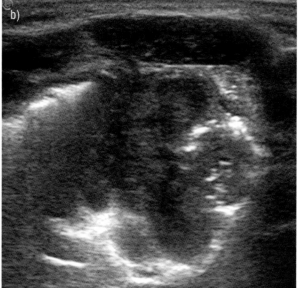

Figure 18.10 **a)** Detail of a larynx X-ray with an endoluminal mass. **b)** Mass ultrasonographic appearance, longitudinal section. The endoluminal gas delimits mass edges.

THYROID GLAND CYSTS (Fig. 18.12–13)

Cystic injuries can be detected in cats with hyperthyroidism (Fig. 18.12), and occasionally in dogs as an incidental finding (Fig. 18.13).

- Changed shape due to simple or septate cysts with hypoechoic-anechoic content
- Irregular edges
- Increased size
- Posterior-wall enhancement.

THYROID GLAND NEOPLASMS (Fig. 18.14–17)

Adenoma and carcinoma of the thyroid can affect canine and feline species. The thyroid adenoma has a decided prevalence in older cats, where it causes thyrotoxicosis. Ultrasonographic features are:

- Unilateral injury in 25 per cent, bilateral injury in 70 per cent, and ectopic injury in 5 per cent of cases
- Rounded shape
- Increased volume (Fig. 18.14)
- Homogeneous to heterogeneous echostructure
- Regular edges
- Cysts may form, giving the gland a complex appearance (Fig. 18.15).

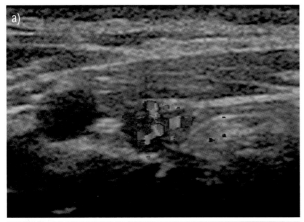

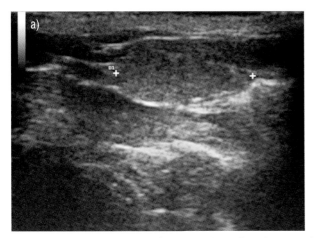

Figure 18.11 Canine hypothyroidism. **a)** Transverse scan of the thyroid, which appears as a hypoechoic and rounded nodule, similar to the carotid artery. The fine vascularization differentiates it from the artery. **b)** Longitudinal scan of the same thyroid lobe. The volume is greatly reduced and the vascularization seems increased; it is actually normal, but the surrounding thyroid tissue is lacking.

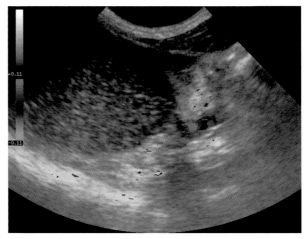

Figure 18.12 Cat; transverse scan performed with a medium frequency microconvex probe of a wide cystic structure located in the left side of the neck. The image shows vascular structures laterally through the colour signal, while the normal gland parenchyma is no longer recognizable. The fluid echogenicity makes it difficult to distinguish the cystic injury from a solid one.

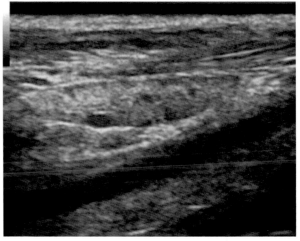

Figure 18.13 Longitudinal scan of a thyroid lobe with microcystic echostructure and decreased subcapsular echogenicity. The figure enables one to identify small anechoic cysts with irregular edges that are diffused throughout the parenchyma; they must not be confused with parathyroid glands and vascular structures.

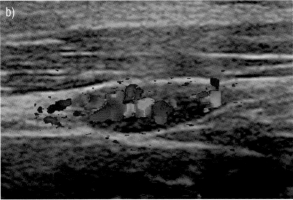

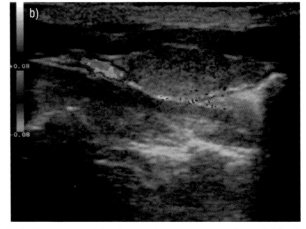

Figure 18.14 Hyperthyroid cat. **a)** Longitudinal scan of an adenomatous lobe. The gland appears rounded and increased in size, characterized by well-defined edges and capsule. **b)** The lobe Colour Doppler highlights the normal intraparenchymal circulation, the carotid artery and the superior thyroid artery.

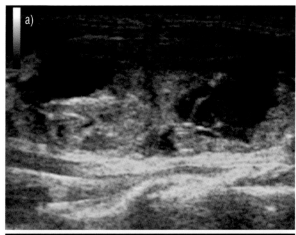

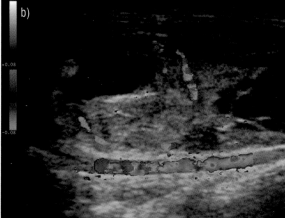

Figure 18.15 Cystic adenoma of the thyroid in a cat with hyperthyroidism. **a)** Longitudinal scan of the left lobe. The gland echostructure is non-uniform due to cystic septate areas with hypoechoic-anechoic content and irregular edges that take up space in the gland parenchyma and contribute to increase in the volume. **b)** The Colour Doppler shows the gland parenchyma vascularization and regional vascular structures. Dorsally to the lobe, the carotid artery is visible.

The thyroid carcinoma mostly affects dogs, and only rarely cats. In most cases it is not secreting, but can induce hypothyroidism, and hyperthyroidism less often. Ultrasonographic features are:

- Unilateral or bilateral injury
- Changed shape due to complex variably sized injuries (mass) (Fig. 18.16a)
- Progressive volume increase
- Hypoechoic heterogeneous echostructure
- Regular or irregular edges and capsule
- Increased, irregular and subcapsular vascularization (Fig. 18.16b and 18.16c)
- Associated changes (vascular and oesophageal invasion, metastases of cervical lymph nodes) (Fig. 18.17).

PARATHYROID GLANDS ULTRASONOGRAPHIC CHANGES

HYPERPLASIA AND ADENOMA

Ultrasonography helps in differentiating hypercalcemic patients suffering from a primary or secondary disease of parathyroid glands (Diagram and Fig. 18.18–20).

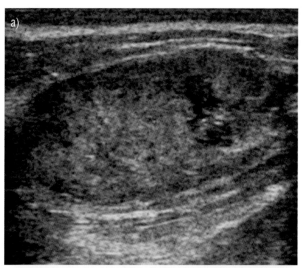

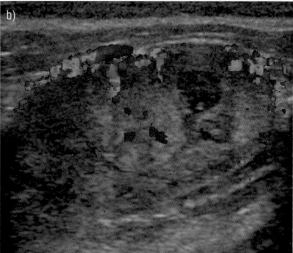

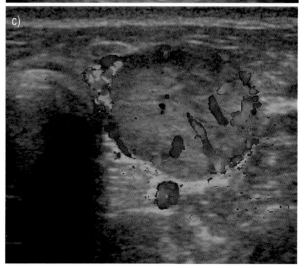

Figure 18.16 Thyroid carcinoma of a dog. **a)** Longitudinal scan, B-mode. The lobe has a heterogeneous echostructure and features a cavitated area with irregular edges and larger than 4 cm in length. **b)** The Colour Doppler of the same carcinoma shows the peripheral distribution of the colour signal that characterizes the strong periparenchymal and intraparenchymal vascularization. The Colour Doppler qualitative analysis allows to integrate B-mode data because the hypervascularization is one of the main malignancy features of the thyroid. **c)** Transverse scan. The Colour Doppler shows that the colour signal is predominantly peripheral and subcapsular. In cross section, the normal flow of the carotid artery is clearly displaced dorsally by the neoplastic lobe size.

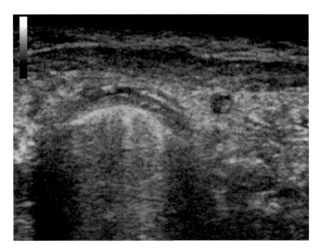

Figure 18.17 Transverse scan of the neck. The image shows the tumour tissue extension at the left carotid artery; the vessel lumen is filled up by echoic structures; in the centre of the image, reverberation artefacts characterize the trachea.

The primary hyperparathyroidism is caused by an adenoma, usually single, and rarely by an adenocarcinoma (Fig. 18.18). The adenocarcinoma is rare and impossible to differentiate from adenomatous nodules, since ultrasonographic features are identical.

The most common secondary form is caused by a chronic renal failure, where all glands can be increased in size (Fig. 18.19).

Ultrasonographic features of a parathyroid nodule are:

- Single nodule, rarely multiple
- Rounded or oval shape
- Increased size, diameter >4 mm

- Hypoechoic-anechoic
- Posterior-wall enhancement
- Well-defined edges.

In malignant hypercalcaemia forms, secondary to a neoplasm secreting the parathyroid hormone-like protein, parathyroid glands are inhibited, then atrophic and reduced to <2 mm in diameter (Fig. 18.20).

RECOMMENDED READING

Rudorf H: Ultrasonographic imaging of the tongue and larynx in normal dogs. Journal of Small Animal Practice. 1997, 38: 439–444.

Reusch CE, Tomsa K, Zimmer C, et al. Ultrasonography of the parathyroid glands as an aid in differentiation of acute and chronic renal failure in dogs. J Am Vet Med Assoc. 2000, 217: 1849–1852.

Hofmeister E, Kippenes H, Mealey KL, Cantor GH, Lohr CV. Functional cystic thyroid adenoma in cat. JAVMA. 2001, 219(2): 190–193.

Reese S, Breyer U, Deeg C, Kraft W, Kasper B. Thyroid sonography as an effective tool to discriminate between euthyroid sick and hypothyroid dogs. J Vet Intern Med. 2005, 19: 491–498.

Bromel C, Pollard RE, Kass PH, Samii VF, Davidson AP, Nelson RW. Ultrasonographic evaluation of the thyroid gland in healthy, hypothyroid, and euthyroid golden retrievers with nonthyroidal illness. J Vet Intern Med. 2005, 19: 499–506.

Radlinsky MG, Williams J, Frank PM, Cooper TC: Comparison of three clinical techniques for the diagnosis of laryngeal paralysis in dogs. Veterinary Surgery. 2009, 38: 434–438.

Tayeman O. K. Peremans K, and Saunders JH. Thyroid Imaging in the Dog: Current Status and Future Directions. J Vet Intern Med 2007; 21: 673–684.

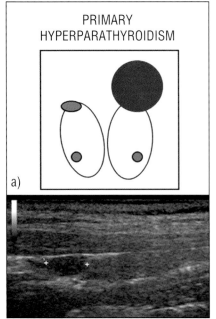

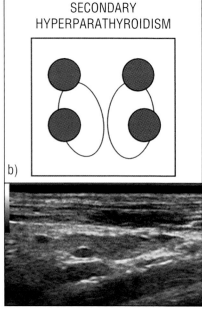

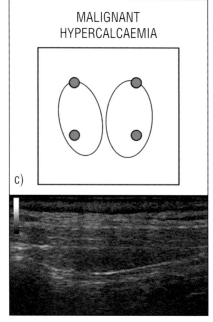

Figure 18.18 **a)** Primary hyperparathyroidism. Sagittal scan of a canine thyroid lobe; the image shows an ipoechoic a nodular injury that warps the cranial pole. The oval morphology, the increased size (8 mm) and the reduction in echogenicity are the ultrasonographic features that characterize parathyroid adenomas. **b)** Secondary hyperparathyroidism. A patient with chronic renal failure. All four parathyroids are increased in volume and prominent. **c)** With malignant hypercalcaemia, parathyroid glands are inhibited and not detectable. Consider however that in a number of healthy patients, parathyroid glands are usually not identifiable.

19 Thoracic ultrasonography

Giliola Spattini

SCAN TECHNIQUE (Fig. 19.1)

Animal preparation	• 12 hours on an empty stomach, at least (essential for retrosternal scans). • Chest hair-clipping, whose extent is determined by the location of the pathological process identified on X-rays. • Hair-clipping at the thoracic entrance. • Parasternal hair-clipping. • Sternal recumbency, right and/or left lateral, quadrupedal posture.
Probes	• Phased-array probe for deeper and movable structures. For surface and not much movable structures, a medium-high-frequency microconvex or linear probe (e.g. 7.5–10 MHz) can be used. • According to the patient size and the depth of the structure to investigate, a 3.5–7.5 MHz probe is used.
Scans and respective probe position	Thoracic entrance scan: • Longitudinal: place the probe (phased-array or microconvex) laterally to the trachea, in the right or left jugular furrow (Fig. 19.1a), tilting it caudoventrally. • Transverse: turn the probe by 90 degrees (Fig. 19.1b). Intercostal scan: • Longitudinal: the head of the probe is positioned over the intercostal space identified by X-ray. The beam is longitudinal compared to the axis of the spine (Fig. 19.1c). • Transverse: the probe is rotated by 90 degrees to obtain a transverse view of the intercostal space (Fig. 19.1d). Parasternal scan: • Longitudinal: the patient is in the lateral recumbency; both sides are investigated: the declivous side and the dorsal one (Fig. 19.1e). In the first case, a table with an opening on the cardiac area is useful. The probe tip is positioned over the apex beat, between the sternum and costochondral junctions. The beam is oriented longitudinally. • Transverse: the probe is rotated by 90 degrees. Retrodiaphragmatic scan (position 7): • Longitudinal: the probe is in contact with the sternum xyphoid process, the beam longitudinally oriented in the cranial direction, with variable obliquity according to the patient chest depth (Fig. 19.1f). • Transverse: the probe is rotated by 90 degrees.

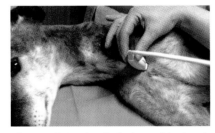

Figure 19.1a Longitudinal scan of the thoracic entrance.

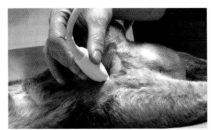

Figure 19.1b Transverse scan of the thoracic entrance.

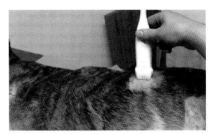

Figure 19.1c Intercostal longitudinal scan.

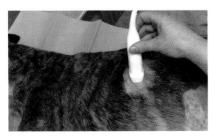

Figure 19.1d Intercostal transverse scan.

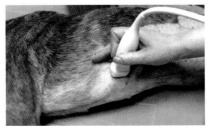

Figure 19.1e Parasternal longitudinal scan, dorsal side.

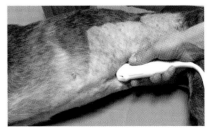

Figure 19.1f Retrodiaphragmatic or retrosternal longitudinal scan.

ULTRASONOGRAPHIC ANATOMY (Fig. 19.2–8)

Location	• Thoracic cavity
Morphology	The chest is a complex region, made by several organs and systems. Usually evaluated structures are: Thoracic wall and rib cage: the following stratigraphy is observed (from outside to inside): • Skin and subcutis: they form a relatively uniform and hyperechoic layer, thanks to adipose and connective tissues (Fig. 19.2). • Intercostal muscles: they form a hypoechoic tissue layer rich in hyperechoic and thin stripes that have a slightly irregular course. • The musculature that is transversal to the first layer has an intermediate echogenicity and accommodates the ribs. Ribs are identified as rounded outlines, with a hyperechoic interface, creating a posterior shadowing. They are regularly distributed and have a curved and smooth surface. Pleura-lung parenchyma interface: • The parietal pleural surface is identified as a well-defined and regular hyperechoic line. The visceral pleura/pulmonary interface is made by an uniform front of reverberation artefact, created by the air within the alveoli (Fig. 19.2). Heart: • It is a moving structure made by echoic walls that encloses a uniformly anechoic content. Both heart chambers and valvular structures are identifiable. Under physiological conditions, the pericardium is impossible to identify (Fig. 19.3). Diaphragmatic interface: • Normally, the diaphragm is not identifiable, unless there is a pleural effusion and a concurrent abdominal effusion. However the lung–liver interface is revealed as an uniform hyperechoic line delimiting the liver and not allowing the visualization of underlying structures. Often a mirror effect artefact is created that shows the liver and gallbladder as if they were deeper than the hyperechoic line (Fig. 19.4). Cranial mediastinum: • On ultrasonography, the cranial mediastinum anatomy is complex. At the thoracic entrance it includes a bundle of blood vessels, some variably sized arterial vessels (usually from three to seven), and the much larger cranial vena cava, located ventrally compared to the arterial bundle (Fig. 19.5). Just ventrally to the vascular bundle, cranial mediastinal lymph nodes are located.
Relationships with adjacent organs evaluable on ultrasonography	• Cranially: goes on with deep fascial planes of the neck region. The thoracic entrance marks the cranial edge of the chest. • Caudally: the diaphragmatic interface delimits the caudal edge of the chest. • Laterally, dorsally, ventrally: the rib cage, the spine and the sternum define the edges of the chest.
Size	Thoracic wall: • The thickness can vary due to adipose tissue deposition. Heart: • The literature reports standard sizes and normality ranges in dogs and cats. Remaining structures are to be valued objectively; a mediastinal shift could witness the increase or reduction in volume of an adjacent thoracic structure.
Edges	Thoracic wall and rib cage: • Wall: smooth and regular edges. Ribs are symmetrically distributed and have a smooth, regular surface. Ventrally, at the costochondral junction, they appear irregular. Pleura–lung parenchyma interface: • Well-defined, smooth and regular edges. Heart: • Well-defined edges, delimited by the pericardium-lung parenchyma interface.

ULTRASONOGRAPHIC ANATOMY (continued)

Edges	Diaphragmatic interface: • Clear and curved edge, often accompanied by a mirror effect artefact. Cranial mediastinum: • Thin, smooth and regular edges.
Echogenicity	Thoracic wall and rib cage: • See the Morphology section. Pleura–lung parenchyma interface: • Very thin hyperechoic line; there is a united front of reverberation artefact. Heart: • Echoic walls, anechoic content. Diaphragmatic interface: • Hyperechoic. Cranial mediastinum: • An echoic tissue surrounds blood vessels and cranial mediastinal lymph nodes (slightly hypoechoic compared to the mediastinal tissue).
Echostructure	Thoracic wall and rib cage: • Fine to coarse. Pleura–lung parenchyma interface • Fine. Heart: • Mean. Diaphragmatic interface: • Fine. Cranial mediastinum: • Mean.
Vessels	Caudal vena cava: • An anechoic tubular structure with a straight course running through the dorsal portion of the liver; it goes past the diaphragm slightly to the right of the midline. With a pleural effusion, it is identifiable up to the outlet into the right atrium (Fig. 19.6). • Similar diameter to the aorta. • Easily compressible lumen; size changes depending on the respiratory phase. Aorta: • It originates from the left cardiac outflow; only a part is evaluable due to the reverberation artefact created by the lung front. Main pulmonary artery: • It originates from the right cardiac outflow; in many patients can be followed up to the bifurcation in the right and left pulmonary artery. Mediastinal vessels: • Identifiable at the thoracic entrance, especially with pleural effusion. Their number can vary. The cranial vena cava is the vessel with the largest diameter and the more ventral location.
Tributary lymph nodes	Cranial mediastinal: • They are located in the cranial mediastinum, just ventrally to great vessels; they may be visible, especially if thickened, either from the thoracic entrance or from a parasternal window (Fig. 19.7). Bronchial: • They are located medially to the bronchi origin of right and left cranial lobes. Under physiological conditions, they are not identifiable on ultrasonography. Hilar • They are located just caudally and dorsally to the bronchi bifurcation of right and left caudal lobes. Under physiological conditions, they are not identifiable on ultrasonography, and often not even in pathological conditions. Sternal: • Just dorsal to the junction between the second and the third sternebra, they are hardly identifiable under physiological conditions, but easily recognizable in case of lymphomegaly (Fig. 19.8).

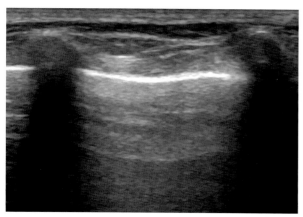

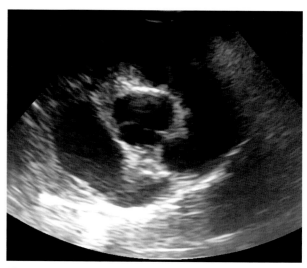

Figure 19.2 Ultrasonographic image of the thoracic wall. Echoic layers (adipose tissue and connective tissue) alternate to hypoechoic layers (muscle tissue). This stratigraphy is broken up by the ribs first, that create a highly absorbent interface: a thin hyperechoic line, and below that a clean posterior shadowing. Then, it is broken up by the visceral pleura–air interface in lungs, where distally to a thin hyperechoic line a wide reverberation artefact follows (dirty posterior acoustic shadow).

Figure 19.3 Transverse image of the heart base. The left atrium (anechoic structure with a stomach-like shape to the right of the image), the aorta and the aortic valve (like the Mercedes symbol), and the right outflow with the opened tricuspid valve are identified. Around the heart, the pulmonary interface creates a uniform echoic area. The pericardium is not identifiable.

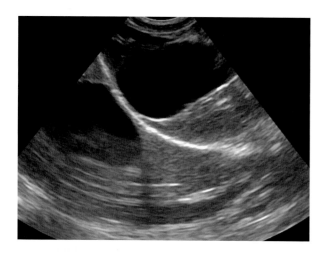

◄ **Figure 19.4** The thin curvilinear hyperechoic interface delimits the liver diaphragmatic aspect and the cranial abdomen. The curvilinear course, the interface between two structures that are very different in acoustic impedance (liver-lung), and the larger size at the ultrasound beam, create a mirror effect artefact: copies of the liver parenchyma and the gallbladder overlap lung fields.

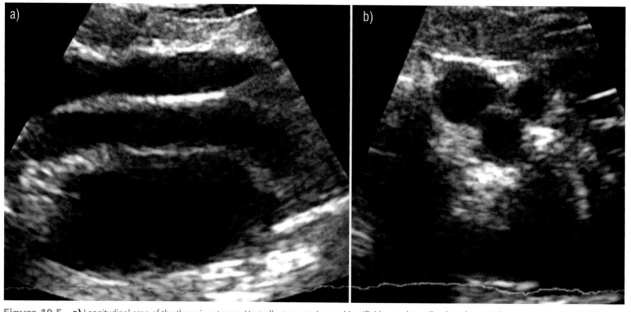

Figure 19.5 **a)** Longitudinal scan of the thoracic entrance. Ventrally, two arteries are identifiable, much smaller than the cranial vena cava that is visible dorsally to those arteries. **b)** Transverse scan of the thoracic entrance: ventrally, three arteries can be identified, while dorsally an oblique scan of the cranial vena cava is visible (anechoic areas). To the left of the arteries, cranial mesenteric lymph nodes are identifiable, if enlarged.

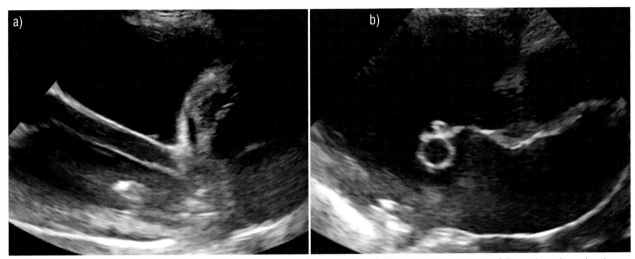

Figure 19.6 **a)** Longitudinal scan of the caudal vena cava in a patient with extensive pleural effusion. The image orientation follows echocardiography rules; so, the caudal portion is to the right of the image, while the cranial portion is to the left of the image (inverted compared to abdominal scans). The vena cava goes past the diaphragm and goes to the right atrium in a straight line. **b)** Transverse scan of the caudal vena cava: it is identified by a well-defined circular structure surrounded by, and connected to, a mediastinal fold.

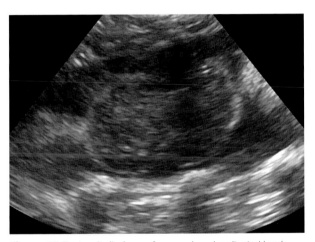

Figure 19.7 Longitudinal scan of a very enlarged mediastinal lymph node in a cat, obtained from a parasternal window. The moderate pleural effusion facilitates the lymph node visualization. The lymph node is so large that it fills the thoracic entrance almost entirely. This is why the lymph node is displaced ventrally until almost touching the sternebrae.

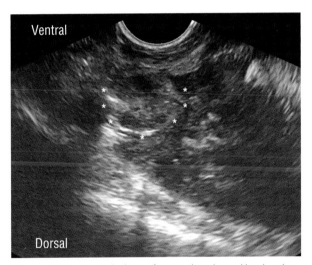

Figure 19.8 Longitudinal scan of a very enlarged sternal lymph node, obtained from a parasternal window. This lymph node has a very ventral position and is located just dorsally to the second-third sternebra.

ULTRASONOGRAPHIC CHANGES

Since the thoracic region is complex and includes several structures, this chapter will be subdivided according to the examined area.

THORACIC WALL

Most common parietal diseases of ultrasonographic interest include:

- Inflammatory diseases
- Foreign bodies
- Neoplastic diseases.

INFLAMMATORY DISEASES (Fig. 19.9–10)

Oedema and cellulitis have a similar ultrasonographic appearance: tissues are thickened and hyperechoic.

While in oedemas tissues tend to maintain well-defined edges, in cellulitis an echoes dispersion is often present, with loss of the normal echostructure.

Seromas and abscesses; they are anechoic collections bounded by a more or less regular and often septate capsule.

- Seromas have an almost completely anechoic content, a very thin and well-defined capsule, and filiform septa
- Abscesses always have a fluid but more echoic content, sometimes layered, with irregular septa and a thick capsule surrounded by hyperechoic tissues with echoes dispersion (Fig. 19.9)
- Small gas infiltrations may be present in thoracic wall tissues, due to a fistulous process that pierces skin tissues, to gas-producing bacteria, or to iatrogenic inoculation (Fig. 19.10).

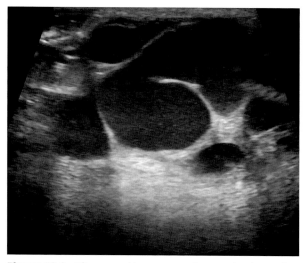

Figure 19.9 Ultrasonographic appearance of an extensive abscess of the thoracic wall. Several sacs are present, containing fluid but rich in echoic foci, bounded by walls and separated by septa. Surrounding tissues are hyperechoic and ill-defined due to the echoes dispersion caused by tissue inflammation.

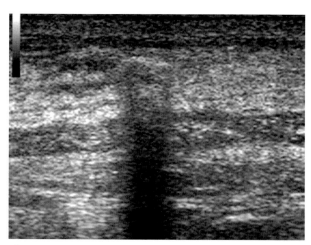

Figure 19.10 A small gas collection within a fistula creates a dirty posterior acoustic shadow; note that the interface is not clear, thin and hyperechoic as generally happens with high acoustic impedance materials; on the contrary, following a not well-defined interface, there is a shadowing rich in echoic foci so that the most superficial portion is echoic. Only in depth, due to the attenuation, does the acoustic shadow become anechoic.

FOREIGN BODIES (Fig. 19.11)

The most common are those of plant origin.

- They have a characteristic lanceolate shape, a pointed end, and a tail formed by very thin ends that diverge from each other (Fig. 19.11)
- They may create a clean posterior acoustic shadow, especially if scanned transversely, where they have a smaller surface but a greater thickness

- Hyperechoic stripes of muscle and adipose tissues may remember a small plant body, but lack the posterior shadowing visible both in longitudinal scans and transverse scans.

NEOPLASTIC DISEASES (Fig. 19.12)

Lipomas have the typical echostructure of the adipose tissue and are well-delimited (Fig. 19.12).

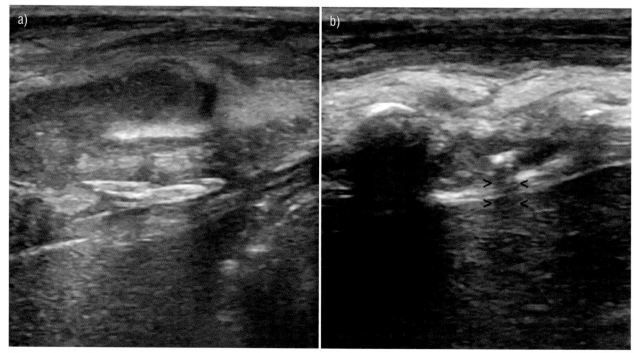

Figure 19.11 a) Longitudinal scan of a plant foreign body. Note the lanceolate appearance. In the longitudinal scan, there is no clean posterior shadowing, probably because of the small thickness of the structure. **b)** In the transverse scan, the foreign body thickness is sufficient to create a clean posterior shadowing (> <) that indicates a material with greater acoustic impedance compared to organic tissues, so it is extraneous with respect to the investigated location. The image shows a rib.

TABLE 19.1	
Features	Description
Size	> size, > chances it is a malignant neoplasm (lipomas excluded)
Echogenicity	The echogenicity is variable, often within the same mass, both in benign and malignant neoplasms
Echostructure	The echostructure tends to be more heterogeneous in malignant neoplasms than in benign ones, due to haemorrhages, mineralizations and necrosis or fibrotic areas
Edges	Edges are often well-defined and regular in benign neoplasms, irregular and difficult to define in malignant neoplasms; however, mast cell tumours tend to have very well-defined edges
Vascularisation	In malignant neoplasms, the vascularization is more disorganized, with more branching than benign neoplasms

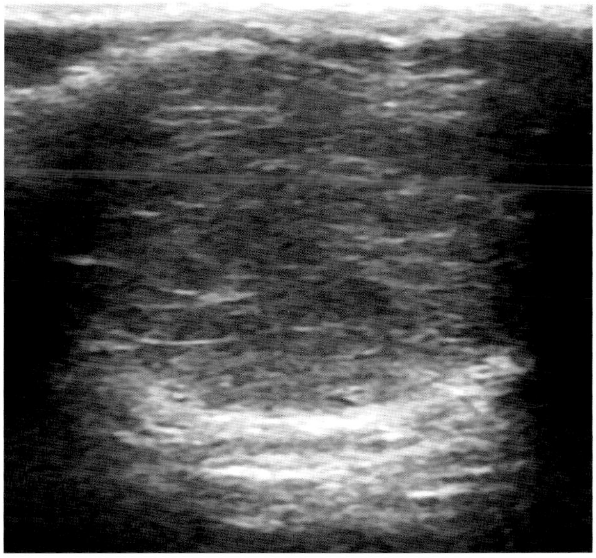

THE PLEURAL EFFUSION (Fig. 19.13–15)

- It is revealed by an anechoic fluid material, which separates the parietal pleura from the lung edges that 'float' in the thoracic cavity (Fig. 19.13)
- The ultrasonographic appearance varies according to the type of fluid. Transudates tend to be completely anechoic, while exudates have fluctuating hyperechoic foci
- Chronic effusions create fibrinous septa that are often thick, irregular and echoic on ultrasonography (Fig. 19.14)
- In case of pyothorax, several saccate collections of fluid material with different echogenicity can be visualized (Fig. 19.15)
- The fluid cytological examination allows for the classification in transudate, modified transudate or exudate.

Pleural nodules are not very common, and mostly often found in mesotheliomas and chronic pyogranulomatous conditions (Fig. 19.16).

- With mesotheliomas, they are usually very small nodules, often hypoechoic, with irregular edges, almost always located at the parietal pleuras. They are found in patients with severe pleural effusion.

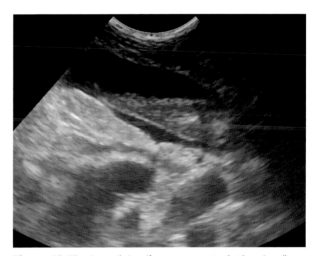

Figure 19.12 Typical ultrasonographic appearance of a lipoma. The echostructure is uniform and hypoechoic, even if hyperechoic compared to the muscle tissue. They have a slightly striated appearance. They have clear and rounded edges, and are bordered by a very thin and well-defined hyperechoic capsule.

Figure 19.13 An anechoic uniform area separates the thoracic wall from a collapsed lung lobe (hypoechoic structure with a triangular shape).

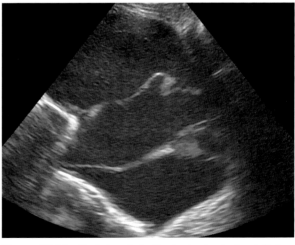

They are almost always recognizable on ultrasonography and differentiable from other neoformations.

Superficial neoplasms can be evaluated on ultrasonography (Tab. 1), even if the final diagnosis always requires a sampling from the injury.

PLEURAE

Most common pleural diseases of ultrasonographic interest include effusion, pleural nodules and pneumothorax.

Figure 19.14 Chest of a patient with extensive chronic pleural effusion. There are irregular echoic septa that cross the chest. The more chronic the effusion, the more the septa tend to be irregular and thickened.

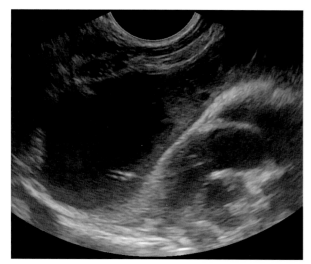

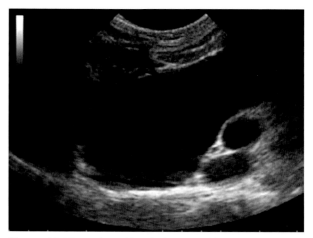

Figure 19.17 Mediastinal branchial cyst in an old cat.

Figure 19.15 Pyothorax in a patient. There is a sac of material with different echogenicity which is in contact with the heart. This sac contains a possibly plant-derived foreign body that can be the pyothorax aetiology.

Among benign injuries, mediastinal cysts must be mentioned, especially common in old cats.

- They are benign injuries which rarely cause respiratory symptoms
- On ultrasonography, they appear as structures stuffed with a fully anechoic material, creating a posterior-wall enhancement, and bounded by a thin and regular echoic wall (Fig. 19.17).

MEDIASTINAL MASSES (Fig. 19.18)

- The most common location of a cranial mediastinal mass is just cranially to the heart, ventrally to the great vessels bundle, more or less ventrally located depending on its size. If very huge, it occupies the whole space from the thoracic entrance up to the heart that can be caudally displaced (Fig. 19.18)
- The lymphoma is the most common mediastinal mass in dogs and cats. The typical ultrasonographic appearance is a hypoechoic nodular mass, with a subtle but clear echoic periphery. It can have different shapes. A Doppler study enables one to visualize the marked vascularization
- The thymoma is an echoic mass with typical cystic injuries that are small and large. However, it can have ultrasonographic features similar to the lymphoma
- Other cranial mediastinum masses to consider in the differential diagnosis are carcinomas originating from ectopic thyroid tissue.

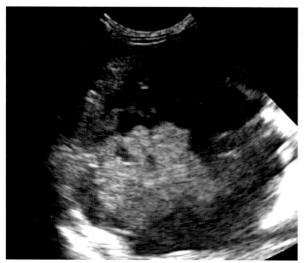

Figure 19.16 Pleural nodule in a patient with mesothelioma.

- Pleural nodules create a mass effect on the lung surface that brush them, but do not move in synchrony with lung movements
- They tend to not invade the thoracic wall towards the outside, but move inward.

With pneumothorax, an air band interposes itself between parietal pleuras and the lung edge. The air band creates a reverberation artefact as if it were the lung surface; however, it does not show synchronous movements with breaths.

MEDIASTINUM

Most common mediastinal diseases of ultrasonographic interest include mediastinal cysts and masses. The mediastinum is a difficult area to investigate both on radiology and on ultrasonography. With a pleural effusion, different acoustic windows open that improve the visualization.

PERICARDIUM (Fig. 19.19)

The pericardial effusion differs from pleural effusion due to the different distribution.

- The anechoic collection is distributed symmetrically around cardiac surfaces
- If there is also a pleural effusion, the thin echoic line representing the pericardium can be visualized; otherwise, an anechoic band surrounding the heart is identified; this is in contact with the hyperechoic interface created by the uniform lung reverberation artefact
- The cardiac tamponade occurs when the intrapericardial pressure is so high as to collapse the right atrium (Fig. 19.19)

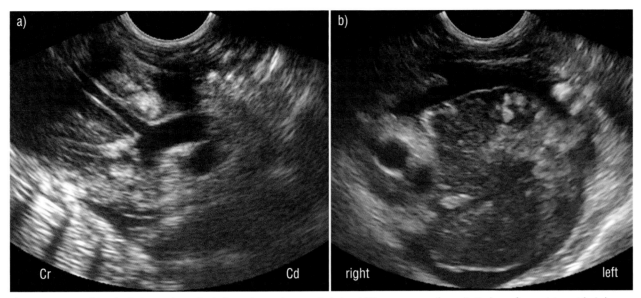

Figure 19.18 **a)** Longitudinal scan of a mediastinal mass from an intercostal window. **b)** Transverse scan of a mediastinal mass from an intercostal window. Mediastinal vessels are partially embedded in the mass.

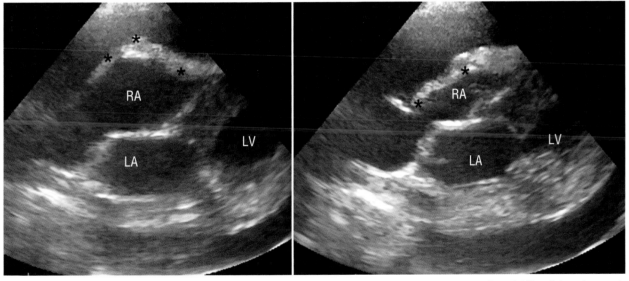

Figure 19.19 A patient with pericardial effusion that collapses the right atrium: in the first image, the right atrium is not collapsed, differently from the second image. The right atrium collapse is the typical ultrasonographic appearance of a cardiac tamponade.

- Before ending the exam, it is recommended to exclude any neoformations, a common aetiology of pericardial effusion
- The most typical location is the heart base.

LUNG (Fig. 19.20–22)

Most common pulmonary diseases of ultrasonographic interest include the collapse, the consolidation, infiltrative diseases and the lung torsion.

On the lung surface, almost all ultrasound waves are reflected from the pleura–lung air interface. This artefact is also called dirty posterior acoustic shadowing.

- If there is a lung disease that alters the gaseous pulmonary contents, this artificial front lacks.

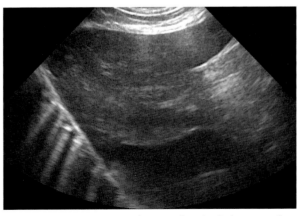

Figure 19.20 Liver–lung interface: cranially to the diaphragm, a uniform mirror effect artefact is usually visible. On the other hand, many comet tails originate from the lung surface. This patient had a pulmonary oedema.

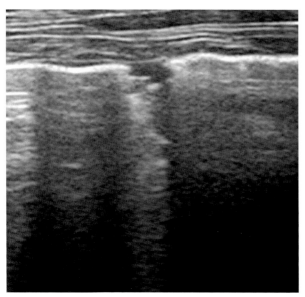

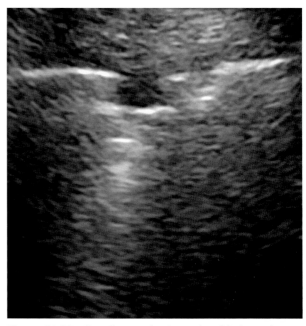

Figure 19.21 The uniform reverberation artefact of the lung surface is interrupted by an injury with ill-defined edges and irregular shape. There is an irregular transition area between the aerated lung and the injury. Comet tails originate from edges of this injury. The appearance is typical of plant foreign bodies' passage.

Figure 19.22 The uniform reverberation artefact of the lung surface is interrupted by a nodular injury with well-defined edges. The nodule has grown compact, moving the aerated tissue gradually laterally and dorsally. The appearance is typical of primary or metastatic lung nodules; usually, a clear boundary is visible between the lung tissue and the neoplastic tissue, and there are no transition areas.

- If there is a modest loss of air from the alveoli, with minimum fluid accumulation or alveolar tissue, the reverberation front is sporadically interrupted by comet tails
- Few comet tails may be normal in a healthy lung, but several tails in the same ultrasonographic image should raise a suspicion of a disease that reduced the alveolar gas content (Fig. 19.20)
- If the lung lesion is small but more defined, as with a small foreign body passage, the injury will be ill-defined, irregularly shaped and surrounded both by hyperechoic foci and comet tails (Fig. 19.21)
- In case of fluid in alveoli, ring-down artefacts increase: in human medicine, ring-downs in lung fields are considered a typical aspect of pulmonary oedema (see Chapter 3, page 17).
- A pulmonary infiltrative process that grows centrifugally and enlarges, gradually removing the air from the alveoli, appears as an injury with well-defined edges, which creates a significant mass effect (Fig. 19.22).

If a pathological process expands to a large area of the lung lobe, the possible findings are pulmonary collapse, consolidation or infiltration.

The collapse or the pulmonary atelectasis occurs every time the air leaves the alveoli, without being replaced by fluids or tissues.

- The lung lobe shows reduced volume, triangular shape and regular and smooth edges (Fig. 19.13)
- The echogenicity depends on the residual air content, and the lung lobe may be uniformly hypoechoic or hyperechoic.

Lung consolidation is caused by all diseases that replace the alveolar air with fluids or cells.

Pneumonia is a common example of lung consolidation.

- Consolidated lung areas can be focal, regional or affecting an entire lobe
- The lung parenchyma is basically hypoechoic
- Typically, the pulmonary anatomy and echostructure remain substantially unchanged, while the volume may be normal or increased
- The bronchi, filled with air, appear as hyperechoic gaseous bronchograms. The air trapped inside creates several reverberation artefacts and comet tails
- When bronchi are filled with fluid or cellular debris, they resemble vessels creating a so-called fluid bronchogram. The consolidated lung reminds one of a liver lobe (Fig. 19.23).

Pulmonary masses can only be identified on ultrasonography if in contact with the diaphragm or the thoracic wall (Fig. 19.24).

- Most lung masses are solid, with a clear mass effect, often showing a mixed echogenicity
- In most cases they do not contain gas. The lung echostructure is changed, and less commonly, gas bubbles remain trapped inside the mass (common finding in inflammatory pulmonary diseases)
- Edges tend to be regular and well-defined, differently to inflammatory processes which typically have irregular and ill-defined edges, rich in comet tail and ring-down artefacts
- Unlike atelectasis and lung consolidation, lung masses usually the normal lung outline.

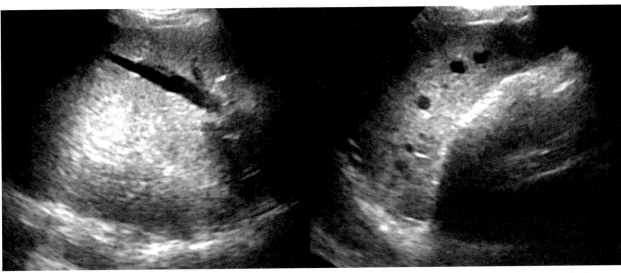

Figure 19.23 Consolidated lung lobe (definitive diagnosis of pneumonia). The lung parenchyma echostructure is fine and echoic. Bronchi contain fluid and remind one of portal vessels (bronchogram liquid).

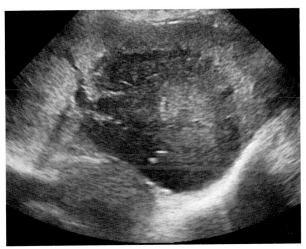

Figure 19.24 A lung mass that originates from a consolidated lung lobe. The mass has well-defined edges, changes the affected lung lobe outline, and the normal lung echostructure is lost. Cytological diagnosis: sarcoma.

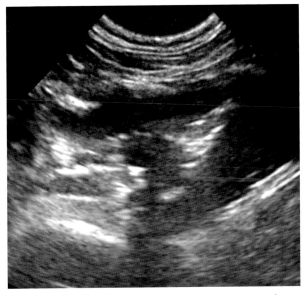

Figure 19.25 Twisted lung lobe. Characteristic signs are scattered hyperechoic foci, with reverberation artefacts concentrated in the central portion of the lung lobe.

Lung metastases are revealed on ultrasonography as:

• Rounded, hypoechoic, peripherally distributed, very well-defined lung nodules compared to the lung reverberation front (Fig. 19.22)
• Often, they appear at the lung–diaphragm interface by altering its profile and reducing the mirror effect. Generally, echostructure and echogenicity of metastases are homogeneous.

LUNG LOBE TORSION (Fig. 19.25)

This is a rare disease, although some breeds are especially predisposed (Greyhounds and Pugs). It is always associated with pleural effusion, even saccate, and it is unclear whether it is a predisposing factor or secondary to the torsion.

Most specific ultrasonographic features are:

• Scattered hyperechoic foci, with or without reverberation artefacts, concentrated in the central area of the lung lobe; this is the more typical ultrasonographic appearance (Fig. 19.25)

• The twisted lobe appears hypoechoic compared to the other lobes, though sometimes full of scattered hyperechoic foci (small gas bubbles in the classic vesicular form)
• Poor or absent vascularization of the twisted lung lobe
• Associated pleural effusion.

DIAPHRAGM (Fig. 19.26–27)

Most common diaphragmatic diseases of ultrasonographic interest are diaphragm rupture (called diaphragmatic hernia) and peritoneopericardial hernia.

DIAPHRAGM RUPTURE

The diaphragm is normally invisible, thus the continuity of the liver–lung interface is not a reliable confirmation of its integrity.

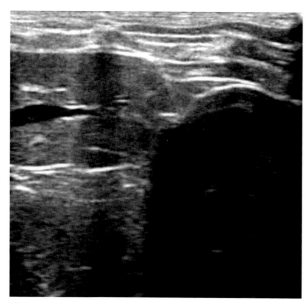

Figure 19.26 In this patient, a liver lobe and a spleen portion are cranial as regards the heart. There is no anatomical separation between the two abdominal and thoracic structures. This is typical of an acute diaphragm rupture.

Artefacts observed at the lung–liver interface may make this diagnosis especially difficult. The ultrasounds refraction can create an uneven liver edge. The mirror effect can mimic abdominal organs in the chest. Moreover, possible hiatuses can create uncertainties.

Most characteristic ultrasonographic signs of diaphragm rupture are:

- Abdominal organs such as the spleen or intestinal loops in the chest (Fig. 19.26)
- The key is to locate the heart and carefully assess its position compared to the liver, the gallbladder and any other organs

- In diaphragmatic hernias, the most often herniated organ is the liver, so it is displaced cranially and the hyperechoic interface that divides it from the heart is lost
- In chronic diaphragmatic hernias, the interface seems to be regular and continuous, due to adhesions between the liver and lung lobes

PERITONEOPERICARDIAL HERNIA

It is a congenital disease caused by the failed completion of the diaphragm that blends into the pericardial sac.

- Abdominal organs are contained in the pericardial sac, in close contact with the heart (Fig. 19.27)
- In case of pleural effusion, the pericardium–pleural effusion interface can be identified.

RECOMMENDED READING

Louvet A, Bourgeois JM: Lung ring-down artifact as a sign of pulmonary alveolar-interstital disease. Veterinary Radiology & Ultrasound 2008. 49: 374–377.

Nyman E, Kristensen AT, Lee MH, Martinussen T, McEvoy FJ: Characterization of canine superficial tumors using gray-scale B mode, color flow mapping, and spectral doppler ultrasonography- A multivariate study. Veterinary Radiology & Ultrasound 2006. 47: 192–198.

Volta Antonella, Mattia Bonazzi, Giacomo Gnudi, Margherita Gazzola, Giorgio Bertoni: Ultrasonographic features of canine lipomas. Veterinary Radiology & Ultrasound 2006. 47: 589–591.

Jung C, Bostedt H: Thoracic ultrasonography technique in newborn calves and description of normal and pathological findings. Veterinary Radiology & Ultrasound 2004. 45: 331–335.

Reichle JK, Wisner ER: Non-cardiac thoracic ultrasound in 75 feline and canine patients. Veterinary Radiology & Ultrasound 2000. 41: 154–162.

Spattini G, Rossi F, Vignoli M, Lamb CR: Use of ultrasonography to diagnose diaphragmatic rupture in dog and cats. Veterinary Radiology & Ultrasound 2003. 44: 226–230.

Zekas LJ, Adams WM: Cranial mediastinal cysts in nine cats. Veterinary Radiology & Ultrasound 2002. 43: 413–418.

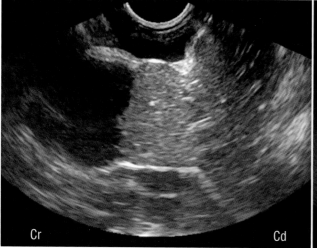
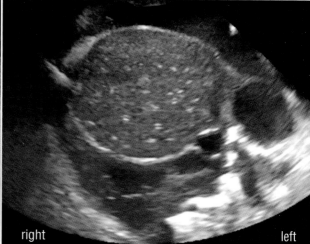

Figure 19.27 Longitudinal and transverse intercostal scan of a cat with pleural effusion secondary to pyothorax. The peritoneopericardial hernia is an accidental finding: the liver is contained in the patient pericardium. Note that, as the liver is within the pericardium, the caudal vena cava and the heart are displaced to the left.

Index

Index